Healthy and Radiant Within

A Prescription for Health
Filled with Inspiring Stories

Best of Health to you!

Sheri Miller

TESTIMONIALS

THANK YOU, THANK YOU for being my greatest inspiration. I renewed my commitment to healthy eating and living and got amazing results. I started feeling fantastic again and I celebrated yesterday by running 10 miles. I feel healthy and powerful again. Miracles in life come in many ways and we need to determine the gift to inspire people. Please don't stop making a difference in peoples' lives! —**Gloria Aliloupour**

Angie and Sheri's book is excellent and full of important information to keep us healthy and free of disease and inflammation. I highly recommend *Healthy and Radiant Within* to anyone interested in living a healthy life. —**Roza Ziemer**

Although I was eating reasonably well when I first read this book, within a very short time, my refrigerator was filled with only good things which I now love to eat. I have no interest in returning to my old eating habits. I also very quickly lost some extra weight around my middle...and my skin looks so clear and refreshed. And strangely, I am eating more enjoyable food than I did before. I now look and feel about 10 years younger and feel so much renewed energy, joy and enthusiasm about my health and body. Thank you, Angie and Sheri! —**Gayna Breedon**

Sheri & Angie's book has given me a strong awareness of the need to eliminate sugars from everyday foods to prevent the long list of diseases. The changes I've made have given me more peace and a sense that I am giving my body what it deserves. I have noticed a big difference in my skin and hair and have been complimented about how good my face and skin look. I find myself much calmer although I lead a hectic life with business and financial deadlines on top of raising two boys with sports every week. My attitude has improved as well as feelings of inner peace. Cheers and be well! —**Adriana Gomez**

Angie and Sheri have not only taught me a whole new way of life, but a whole new state of mind. It has been their passion, and sharing what they know and have experienced, that has me much happier and aware. —**Marvida Rodriguez**

Years of combined experience have made Angie and Sheri experts in their own health and healing. Their inspired wisdom is sure to empower countless others on their own path to wellness and self-discovery. —**Noreen Auterio Scoggins**

Thanks, Angie and Sheri! I have started being so much more conscious of the amount of sugar my family and I are consuming. Wow, it is crazy how easy it is to eat a lot of sugar! So I'm taking baby steps, albeit baby steps, to cut that down considerably. With gratitude! —**Ursula Hawe**

Healthy and Radiant Within is extremely impressive with the amount of useful information, inspiring stories and knowledge these two women share. I thought I knew a lot about the subject of health and wellness, but I came away with much more than I anticipated! I highly recommend this book! —**Julie Yip**

I suffered from stomach and digestion problems and it was Angie and Sheri who made me realize the connection between my diet and well-being. THANK YOU SO MUCH for enlightening me on my health when even a doctor of gastroenterology couldn't. —**Ed Rickles**

Healthy and Radiant Within

A Prescription for Health
Filled with Inspiring Stories

Angie Lambert
&
Sheri Miller

Healthy and Radiant Within: A Prescription for Health Filled with Inspiring Stories

ISBN-13: 978-1984132277
ISBN-10: 198413227X

Available from Amazon.com and other online stores

Disclaimer: This book is intended as a practical guide for anyone, healthy or unhealthy, stressed or in pain, who seeks to transcend his or her limitations. Dietary or lifestyle advice in this book is not a replacement for medical treatment but can be a vitally important complement toward healing, wholeness and well-being. Please consult with a doctor who specializes in your condition before solely trying these recommendations.

DEDICATION

Angie:
To my lovely daughter, Alana

Sheri:
*To my dear children and grandchildren,
may you be well and thrive.*

CONTENTS

FOREWORD

Lifestyle is the most powerful medicine on the planet. Doesn't it make sense then to pay attention to the style in which we live our lives?

In their book, *Healthy and Radiant Within: A Prescription for Health Filled with Inspiring Stories,* Angie Lambert and Sheri Miller have assembled forty-five personal stories that describe simple, effective and powerful ways to transform disease to optimal health using lifestyle modification strategies. Each of their stories involves real people with real illnesses that are wonderful examples of why they became ill and what they did to recover and feel good again.

The strategy the authors endorse embraces a hierarchy of treatment modalities that for the sake of safety, effectiveness, and cost dictates that the least invasive therapy should be utilized first whenever possible. Lifestyle strategies such as diet, exercise, adequate sleep, stress reduction, weight control, avoidance of toxic exposures, and securing emotional and spiritual balance in life are the first line of defense. Natural medicine approaches based on the latest advances in orthomolecular medicine and functional medicine are the next line of defense. Noninvasive Complementary and Alternative Medicine (CAM) services such as acupuncture, herbal medicine, chiropractic, bodywork, homeopathy, and energy medicine are next in line of defense. Very careful and sparing use of pharmaceutical drugs, surgery, and other invasive strategies are the very last line of defense.

Lambert and Miller advocate a paradigm shift that embraces wellness as the primary goal. These authors point out that there is something more that goes beyond lifestyle as a way of promoting radiant health. They have made the extraordinary point to consider the role of spirituality in health and disease.

This book focuses on a model of nutrition, environment, and stress as the basis for causing most diseases and on solutions anchored in functional medicine approaches. It is an excellent comprehensive review of a multitude of health conditions that is easy to read and filled with commonsense solutions that are safe, effective, affordable, and doable.

Sadly, today's health care is primarily a business, not a service. It is based on a sick care model that profits when we are sick and goes bust when we're healthy. Health care businesses are responsible to their stockholders whose bottom line is return on their investment. Treatment is not necessarily oriented to doing what is best to restore and maintain excellent health for patients, but on approaches that generate the most income.

It is important to realize that the greater the cost of health care the greater the profits generated by the health care industry. Big pharma, the insurance industry, doctors, hospitals, medical technology, and medical research all depend on spending more of our money to make more for themselves. If you want to understand how today's health care model works, follow the money!

The authors challenge the concept of waiting until we get sick before seeking health care. This outdated model gives lip service to wellness and prevention, with its focus on fixing our ailing health after it has gone south.

The underlying message here is that if you are dealing with a health challenge, this book will save you time and money on the road to being healthy and radiant. ◆

—Len Saputo, MD

Bio

Len Saputo, MD, graduated from UC Berkeley and Duke University Medical School. Board certified in Internal Medicine, he was in private practice at John Muir Medical Center from 1971 to 2004. Dr. Saputo is a pioneer in bridging the gap between mainstream and Complementary and alternative medicine. He is the founder of the Health Medicine Forum, a nonprofit educational foundation, the Health Medicine Center, and co-founder of the Health Medicine Institute for Research. Dr. Saputo is a motivational speaker, radio show host with his wife Vicki, and the author of many books and articles.

Among other publications and papers, Dr. Saputo is the author of *A Return to Healing—Radical Health Care Reform and the Future of Medicine* with Byron Belitsos.

Acknowledgments

We would like to express our heartfelt appreciation to the following individuals who contributed to *Healthy and Radiant Within.*

Andrea Hurst, Marie De Haan, and Barbara Hyde for their skillful editing work.

Patricia G. Linden and Joni Wilson, for their expertise in formatting this book.

Deborah Perdue, Illumination Graphics, for designing our radiant book cover.

Thank you to our generous story contributors who share their personal healing journeys and remind us that the power to heal always was and is within each of us.

Love and gratitude to medical pioneer Len Saputo, MD, for writing the foreword to this book.

INTRODUCTION
OUR "WHY" FOR WRITING THIS BOOK

Every day is another chance to get stronger
to eat better
to live healthier
and to be the best version of you.

Having overcome chronic illnesses ourselves, we are compelled to tell our stories and feel a responsibility to share what we have learned. This book is about triumph over illness and mastery of oneself in the process. The 45 personal stories in this book, ranging from diabetes to cancer to heart disease, illustrate how individuals dramatically changed their lives through discipline and determination.

Our intention is to provide hope and alternatives not widely promoted in our Western culture. The maintenance of our health begins with the lifestyle choices you and I make every day. Our daily choices contribute to good health or to the deterioration of our health. The choice is ours. Food and thought are the two things we can control. Self-mastery over both is key and allow us to live our lives with purpose and vitality.

We believe healing from chronic disease is about transformation, and can be an avenue for personal and spiritual growth. Our bodies are talking to us and when we get desperate enough, we begin to listen. Reclaiming one's health is not merely a physical journey. There is more to illness than a diagnosed disease. There are stories our soul wants to tell us, lessons our being wants us to learn. If our life becomes taking pills for every problem and challenge, then perhaps we miss the insight our body is trying to give us.

Our health is the interaction of all facets of our lives: from our genetics to diet, exercise, thoughts, emotions, relationships, jobs, environment, and more. When we are willing to look more closely at the nature of our choices, we can begin to take responsibility for our health and well-being.

Many of us got the message throughout childhood that doctors were the authority and we deferred to them to be the experts of our bodies. Over time, many people have discovered there's more to healing than popping pills or following "doctor's orders."

Many physicians are not adequately trained to determine the underlying causes of complex, chronic diseases. Their education doesn't include applying strategies such as nutrition, exercise, and lifestyle changes to prevent and treat the illnesses in their patients.

At times traditional medical treatment such as drugs and surgeries are a necessity. But prescription drugs have become the norm and a widely accepted way of life for both adults and children. Many of us are needing other options we aren't getting. This book you are holding offers you information and stories to bridge the gap and provide alternative choices and the education piece that is often missing.

Fortunately, there are medical doctors and practitioners who follow an integrative and preventive approach to health who emphasize nutrition and lifestyle for managing and reversing chronic disease. A few of our favorites include Dr. Mark Hyman, Dr. Len Saputo, Dr. Nancy Appleton, Dr. Bruce Lipton, Ann Louise Gittleman, Dr. Joel Fuhrman and Dr. Andrew Weil. We will refer to them throughout this book.

As best-selling author Dr. Mark Hyman states in his book, *The Blood Sugar Solution*, "When you take out the bad stuff and put in the good stuff, the body knows what to do and creates health. Disease goes away as a side effect of creating health."

Throughout this book, we offer tips to assist you in being more mindful about your daily choices, regardless of the challenge you are facing. Mindfulness is simply paying attention in the present moment, which can ultimately help us make healthier decisions.

How we perceive and think about our experiences determine how we respond to stress, pain, and illness. The latest DNA research illustrates that by changing your perception, your mind can alter the activity of your genes and create over thirty thousand variations of products from each gene. In the simplest terms, this means that we need to change the way we think if we are to heal.

Research from the University of California, San Francisco, by E. Epel and E. Blackburn, shows that stressful thoughts and worry influence the rate at which we age, down to our cells and our DNA. We know that stress is a major player in health and disease. We share ways to handle stress and include a variety of alternative therapies to consider.

Our personal journeys back to health required patience and discipline. It's our privilege to teach what we learned to assist you on your journey. If you are dealing with a health challenge, consider us your health guides on your road to wellness. We're here to save you time, frustration and visits to your medical doctor for endless prescriptions that mask symptoms without addressing root causes. A health challenge can be a lonely experience; we want you to know you're not alone.

It is our hope that as you tap into your inner physician and align with your body's wisdom and intelligence, you will have a greater chance to heal yourself. By paying attention to the wisdom of your body and the power of your choices, you can experience radiant health.

Chapter 1
Our Journeys Back to Health

Difficult roads often lead to beautiful destinations.

Journey Back to Health—Angie L.

My passion for running began as a young girl growing up in a small town in South Dakota. I loved all sports, and in high school won state championships in track and cross country. While at Minnesota State University, I earned All-American status in indoor track. Then I met a man, fell in love, and transferred schools. The relationship was controlling and unhealthy. I was working full time and attending school full time. As a result of my schedule and my relationship, I felt stressed. Within a few months, I began having aches and pains all over my body. Finally I could barely get out of bed. I went to the doctor who gave me exercises to do and made me feel like it was all in my head. Weeks later, at my mother's insistence, I went to the emergency room at the University of Minnesota Hospital, and my blood was tested. I was diagnosed with rheumatoid arthritis. I was twenty years old.

The news was devastating. I soon left my unhealthy relationship and my pain and inflammation immediately got fifty percent better. I continued to treat my condition with prescription Motrin, cortisone shots, and later, surgeries to correct joint deformities. In my late twenties, I went to see a well-known and well-respected rheumatologist and board chairman for the National Arthritis Foundation, Dr. Rodney Bluestone. After reviewing my X-rays, he told me, "At the rate your joints are degenerating, you'll be in a wheelchair by forty." He said my joints were "wearing away like an eraser on a pencil." At that moment I did not know where to turn.

For the next decade, I continued to have joint pain mostly in my hands and feet, with difficulty walking and even driving, crawling up and down stairs because it was too painful to walk. I took a long list of prescribed medications (Imuran, Methotrexate, Vioxx, and Celebrex) in addition to over-the-counter pain meds. I was on six 800 mg of prescription Motrin, equivalent to twenty-four over-the-counter Motrin to comfortably get through the day. I limped each morning to walk until my meds kicked in. Strangers would ask, "Are you ok?" I replied, "Yes, thanks. I'm just waiting for my pain meds to kick in."

Once, while getting my monthly blood test, a male lab technician confided in me. He said, "You're too young to be taking these meds. I see the lab results. Do whatever you can to get off these drugs. Don't tell them I told you."

The lab tech was an angel in disguise. He was my wake-up call.

Months later, I was working at a computer company with one of my best friends Amy, who came into the office very excited to share news with me. Amy had taken a walk that morning with a woman who shared her story about having arthritis and reversing it with diet. She told Amy she gave up flour, dairy, and sugar and had amazing results. Amy said, "It can't hurt to try it." Another angel in disguise. Luckily, I was paying attention.

I began monitoring my diet and immediately noticed when I steered away from foods containing flour, dairy, and sugar, my joints felt better! I saw a direct relationship between certain foods and inflammation. Giving up products made with white or wheat flour had a *profound* positive impact on my health and healing. Today, we know those flour products contained gluten.

I read books on arthritis (such as *The Arthritis Cure*) and took glucosamine and chondroitin. Eventually, I gave up coffee, then finally Diet Coke, and eventually all artificial sweeteners. I started receiving acupuncture treatments a couple times a week. Those needles felt like they popped mini balloons of inflammation.

A turning point for me was my parents introduced me to a woman who had gotten out of a wheelchair by taking a nutritional supplement. I began taking this supplement, and within a few weeks it gave me more mobility and ease in my body.

As I came into more mind and body awareness, I learned to meditate, discovered a wonderful non-denominational church, and participated in a study group called A Course in Miracles. As I engaged in these practices, I experienced more freedom in my body.

My efforts paid off. I went from limping, to walking, to jogging again. In spite of Dr. Bluestone saying I would be in a wheelchair around that time of my life, I completed the Honolulu Marathon, fulfilling a childhood dream to one day run a marathon.

In Honolulu, I was awarded "Outstanding Team Member" by the National Arthritis Foundation (NAF) and was asked to be a spokesperson for future marathon participants involved with the foundation.

Through research, discipline, and determination, I am completely pain-free and have been for several years. By changing my diet, eliminating offending foods, and learning to be more mindful, my body came back into balance.

I continue to be very conscious of how I eat and care for myself. If I ingest too many "inflammatory" foods, I may experience a tiny bit of joint discomfort. As soon as I get back on my program, I am again pain-free.

Today, I feel better than I ever dreamed of in my twenties. I am a single mom, raising a young daughter who is the love of my life. I'm so grateful I have the health and energy to keep up with her!

Have faith, and let feeling good and being healthy be your motivation. ♦

Lyme Disease: My Gift of the Wound—Sheri M.

As I trimmed shrubs on a warm and sunny Tuesday afternoon on April 11, 1993, what was about to happen would change my life forever.

I was newly divorced and getting my house ready to put on the market when I noticed the shrubs in front of the house needed trimming. Wearing shorts and wielding large pruning shears, I chopped until I was pleased with the results. Now it was time to prepare the garage sale.

As I gathered items to sell, I noticed a slight rash on my left thigh but didn't think too much about it. The next morning, I applied poison oak cream thinking I might have brushed against a poison oak bush. The rash remained and by the next day, the joints in my wrists ached. By the weekend, I ran a fever and felt like I had the flu.

After nearly a week with flu-like symptoms, I called my doctor and was told to come in the following week if I wasn't feeling better. In the meantime, I decided to do some research on my own as I wondered if the rash and the flu symptoms were connected. At the time, the Internet was not yet a commonly used tool for research, so I ordered a hot topic file on infectious diseases from a medical research company. I spent the weekend pouring over the information and by Monday morning, I suspected that I might have Lyme disease.

My doctor agreed to run a blood test for Lyme and the tests came back inconclusive. As a precautionary measure, she put me on three weeks of antibiotics. I started feeling better and moved forward with selling my house. The rash and symptoms were blips on the screen of life.

Fast forward two years: I now lived in a new condo, happily fixing it up and getting used to being single. But my body was not quite right. I had pain in my left hip area, and my energy level wasn't what it should be. I chalked it up to adjusting to my new life, but as the symptoms worsened, I returned to the same doctor that I had seen two years previously. She tested me for various illnesses that can cause fatigue: Epstein-Barr virus, anemia and fibromyalgia. When none of these seemed to fit, she referred me to an infectious disease doctor. This new doctor could find nothing wrong. Still no diagnosis.

Fast forward seven years: I visited at least eight different doctors but still had no diagnosis. My fatigue had worsened, and I could no longer exercise. This was very disconcerting, as I had always done aerobics and tried to keep in shape.

I also had pain and stiffness in my neck. My eyes tired easily and my vision blurred. I had brain fog and my ability to remember things slipped. I'm not normally prone to depression, but I felt disheartened and discouraged.

I decided to start a chronic fatigue support group. I made flyers and distributed them at a health forum meeting. Within a short time we formed a small group and began to share stories and offer support to one another. One of the women got diagnosed with Lyme disease by a specialist in San Francisco. I visited the same doctor and together with my blood tests and clinical symptoms discovered I, too, had Lyme disease.

Finally, a diagnosis!

I was put on antibiotics again, but after two years, my body couldn't handle them anymore. I felt a little better but continued experiencing debilitating symptoms. I stopped working as a speech therapist as I could no longer sit without pain for extended periods of time. My ability to plan lessons and work with students greatly diminished. I turned to alternative medicine and began working with a naturopathic doctor. I changed my diet, took supplements, meditated, practiced gentle yoga, and prayed. I learned about John of God, a healer in Brazil, and took a long journey to see him.

I also started using the Rife machine. Vibrations emitted through electrodes shattered the spirochetal lyme bacteria cell wall. At first I was skeptical when hearing about this technology. But antibiotics weren't curing me, and I didn't want to leave any stone unturned.

Of all the approaches I tried, changing my diet brought the most positive changes to my healing process. I discovered that when I eliminated sugar and gluten and cut back on dairy, I felt much better. My head was clearer and I had more energy. Over time, eating consciously became a natural part of my life. In addition to feeling better, being able to choose fresh, wholesome foods helped me feel I had more control over my illness.

Although I dealt with this debilitating disease for many years, today I lead a full life as a Health Coach, working with children as a speech therapist, and enjoying my kids and grandchildren. I have embraced a more mindful way of living and thinking, and life has taken on a sweet appreciation that previously wasn't there.

What an experience it has been to be humbled by an insect no bigger that the size of a pinhead. But my life has given me the opportunity to learn that I have inner strength, courage, and determination that I might never have had the chance to experience without this health challenge.

This revelation I have come to call the Gift of the Wound. ◆

Psoriasis, My Greatest Teacher—Angie L.

I was 18 years old and in my freshman year of college when my scalp began to itch. The long hours of sitting and studying seem to accumulate nervous energy that manifested as excess skin scales on my scalp. So I bought special shampoos to calm it down. This helped.

I didn't think much about my scalp condition until it showed up a couple years later on my elbows, knees, fingers and toes. I did what every good American does with a skin issue and scheduled an appointment to see a dermatologist. I sought out a top medical doctor who, at the time, was Dr. Nicholas Lowe in Santa Monica. He prescribed pills and UV light along with various steroid topical creams. And so my psoriasis journey began.

Each week in my 20s, I visited Dr. Lowe's office, waiting for my name to be called, to join several other psoriasis patients who stripped down in tent-like booths, took pills, lathered up in lotion and stood in front of U-V light for anywhere from 15 seconds to a couple minutes. The light was a way of suppressing the skin cells and slowing down their duplication, since psoriasis is a condition where skin cells reproduce at 30 times the normal rate, causing skin cells to accumulate, turn white and became itchy, red and inflamed.

After a few years of this type of light treatment, I resorted to tanning booths which was less bothersome than going to a doctor's office. So I kept the skin somewhat under control by being very tan and using topical steroid creams and lotions. I began to get acupuncture twice a week and this seemed to provide even more relief. Still, it was all a bandage for real, long-term healing. When I eased up on the sessions, back came the psoriasis.

I read books like *Healing Psoriasis* by Jon O.A. Pagano which was inspiring and instilled hope. I tried all of his approaches, working with a chiropractor on specific areas of spinal adjustments. I went off refined sugar, got off wheat (gluten), tomatoes and coffee. (I was gluten free long before it became the current trend.) My diet helped the skin be less itchy and inflamed, but still, there it was.

I met various people who healed their psoriasis. But no one seemed to do it the same way. I tried flax seed oil, primrose oil and a zillion other supplements over the years—both topical and internal. I made my own kombucha tea with a live mushroom 20 years before Whole Foods sold bottled kombucha tea.

I knew emotions were connected to having this skin condition. There was a period of two years I was extremely happy and the psoriasis seemed to disappear during this time. But when it came back, it did so with a vengeance. Especially after a break up with a boyfriend. I wondered, how could I duplicate that happiness and get the positive result again?

I got married in my 30s and we moved to the Bay Area, San Francisco. My skin was still an issue so I sought out Dr. John Koo of San Francisco, known as the "Psoriasis Guru." I decided to be part of a skin study for psoriasis, taking pills and doing light treatments three times a week for three months. It was a big-time commitment but the treatment was completely free. I wasn't sure if I was receiving the real treatment or a placebo. I watched my skin clear and get tan from the light and felt great about myself again. I found out I was in fact taking the real drug that amplified the effect of UV light. So I continued on with that treatment until I got tired of commuting to the city.

A few months later, the psoriasis came back. All the suppression unleashed a major outbreak. I was beyond frustrated. I was allowing psoriasis to affect my self-esteem and happiness. Here I was teaching classes on nutrition as a health coach, leading tai chi and meditation classes for relaxation, but underneath my clothes my skin was a mess. I was perplexed, yet still determined.

I learned about a tar treatment through UCSF San Francisco whereby a patient spends 5-6 weeks in scrubs, covered in tar and plastic for the entire day Monday through Friday as a "hospital" day patient. If the patient is lucky, she or he is clear of psoriasis for anywhere from one year up to 10 years after the tar treatment is completed. So with good insurance, I registered to be a "tar patient" at what I called the "tar pit" through UCSF Psoriasis Clinic in San Francisco under Dr. John Koo and his interns.

So off I went each day into the city. To undress, get covered in tar and plastic, put on hospital scrubs. In addition patients received UV light treatment each day as well. So there we all sat together — those of us suffering with severe psoriasis, talking, watching movies together, reading books, sharing our stories, hoping our time spent at the "tar pit" would prove to be successful and provide long-term relief.

I put in my 5 1/2 weeks. Upon completing the tar and light program, my skin was again tan and healthy...and I felt amazing...for six months. Some people got *years* of clear skin after this tar treatment. I got six months. Then all the psoriasis returned, again.

So I did more research and found a doctor close to home. I set up an appointment with Dr. Robert Greenberg, who was a well-known dermatologist specializing in psoriasis in San Ramon, CA. His office had light booths but he also prescribed the new biological drugs that target auto immune conditions such as psoriasis.

I hated the idea of doing self-injections. But I was desperate. I wanted to focus on being a Holistic Health Coach supporting clients without the distraction of a skin disorder and the itching, flaking and frustration that accompanied it.

Throughout these years I asked the deeper questions to myself about what the psoriasis was really about and what it was here to teach me. I got hints and clues along the way, but clearly I was still missing a piece of the puzzle. It was ironic for me to be a believer in holistic approaches and solutions when I myself could not seem to find the ultimate answer to my health dilemma.

After doing a lot of research, I made a decision to try Humira, the biologic drug that balances out an overactive immune system by suppressing it. Yes, even with all of the potential (lethal) side effects, I reached a point where I was willing to try anything that would provide relief and not be as time consuming as other treatments. I decided I would rather risk dying from a biologic drug than live with this annoying, distracting, unsightly, messy, painful skin disease.

I received my first double injection of Humira into both legs in Dr. Greenberg's office. It was challenging to find a clear spot of skin where the nurse could inject. I cried. But not because it hurt. Because I was so desperate, so frustrated, so uncomfortable and yet hopeful that this drug could actually help me. From that day forward I would do a self-injection every two weeks.

Three weeks after the first double injection, my skin was completely clear, smooth, normal. I was free. I felt happy. I could be present for my clients. I could be confident again. I could feel normal and healthy again. I gave thanks and praise to the inventor of this drug, despite being a holistic-minded health coach who taught others how to heal without drugs and medical intervention. Humira was not a cure. But I was grateful.

So every two weeks I gave myself an injection, switching legs each time. My skin remained clear but I remained fearful of what could happen suppressing my immune system with this drug. The list of potential side effects was very long. In time I would inject only monthly to reduce my risk. My skin still stayed clear.

I remained on Humira until the end of 2015 and then stopped cold turkey. I was done. I had gone through a divorce and had done a lot of emotional healing and I wanted to see what happened if I went off the drug.

As the days and weeks went by, my skin began to be covered in scales, redness, itching and inflammation. I just allowed it to be there. Accepted it. Embraced it. Sent it love and light. I am spiritual and am aware that love is the greatest healer. But somehow that still wasn't enough.

I had spent the previous eight years taking workshops and classes to learn about energy and energy healing techniques. I studied and practiced a healing modality called Spiritual Response Therapy (SRT) and spent years doing "clearings" to get to the bottom of my psoriasis. I received clues about the root cause. My search for a cure continued.

I worked with gifted healers and learned about myself and how I "run my energy." I learned I had "soft boundaries" energetically speaking, allowing others into my energy field. I learned I was an "appeaser," pleasing others at my own expense.

At some point in my life I stopped aligning with my own truth in order to be what others wanted and needed. The cost was high. I stopped believing in myself or knowing who I really was.

I learned that I was taking on other people's energy and then my body had to process all that unwanted energy. I had to change this pattern, this "energy dance."

I had to learn to have firm boundaries with others both energetically and in my relationships. I had to learn to say no and speak my truth. I had to get to the core of my low self-esteem, which didn't make any sense to me. I had a fun childhood, excelled in sports, got good grades, had close friends and was a happy person, despite my health challenge.

I was so determined to heal myself and my skin. I was committed to loving myself, but I didn't know how.

I enrolled in a 13-week course led by Katie Macks. It was a deep dive into uncovering unconscious, self-limiting beliefs. I had a lot of them. Untruths that ran my life. Hidden beliefs that kept me playing small. A critical mind that kept me from truly loving myself.

Throughout these 13 weeks, I was able to uncover my "stories" and limiting beliefs that life wasn't safe. After all, others can hurt you. I didn't fear physical harm as much as emotional and energetic harm. So I covered myself in psoriasis to keep me safe and separate from others. Psoriasis was my false sense of safety and security.

Three highly conscious, loving women took Katie's powerful course with me and reflected back to me truths that helped me uncover and break through ways of being that no longer served me. They, along with Katie, supported me in reconnecting to my authentic self.

Finally, I was able to see what soft boundaries and appeasement tendencies had cost me. I assured myself I was safe and lovable, with or without psoriasis. There was fear about being my authentic self. Would people still love me if I wasn't jumping through hoops to please them? If I stopped being an easy going "yes girl"? If I stopped giving so much of myself?

It was time to return to my authentic self. Time to speak my truth. To BE my truth. To create firm boundaries with others. To say "no" if something didn't feel right. To move away from unhealthy relationships. To say "yes" to me, my life, my love for myself. To realize my own value, my contribution and my goodness. To let go of self-criticism once and for all and own my true worth.

As I learned to own my worth, I could more easily embrace myself with love, kindness, gentleness, compassion and acceptance. To stand boldly in my truth and have enough respect for myself that I no longer felt the need to appease and over-please others. This was a huge relief.

Now, if I'm going to do a generous or kind act, I ask myself, "Is this coming from true joy and my heart or is this appeasement, to please another so they like me or approve of me or don't get upset with me?" If it's the latter, I don't do the thing I was thinking about doing.

If I see something beautiful and inspirational and ask myself, "Who should I buy this for?" I listen to the still, small voice that replies, "You." I smile and say to myself, "Yes, this is for me." Then I buy it and enjoy the beauty and inspiration it brings me. Without guilt. Because it's okay to love ourselves and treat ourselves with love, kindness and generosity. It's not selfish, it's essential.

I'm no longer afraid of direct communication or being honest with myself or another. I have less fear about what others think. I see my potential more clearly now. My vision is bigger than I could ever see when I was busy pleasing others and ensuring people liked me or approved of me. I now tune in to what's right for me and that informs my decision-making.

It took 30 years, but today I have clear, healthy skin...without light, without creams, without pills, without tar, without injections. I am attuned with the truth of my soul. I am on my path. I am aligned with Spirit/Source/God/Universe and my Angels. And I have clear, healthy boundaries with others.

Healing comes when we are willing to stop and pay attention to all of our innate body's messages and wisdom. It has so much to teach us.

Psoriasis has been my greatest teacher. I'm grateful for all it has taught me. I'm thankful I didn't give up. I'm happy for all I learned in my quest to heal my skin.

The ultimate message it had for me? To love, honor, and respect myself. To have kindness and compassion for myself. I always had it for others, but I lacked it for myself. I have learned to see and live the truth of my being.

When I stand in this place, all is well. I am safe. To the extent I love myself, I can love all of life. To the extent I love myself, I teach my daughter to love herself, too. Each of us affects the whole.

Love is the greatest healer. But sometimes we have to take the time to see what's in the way of love for self, follow our inner guidance and make the necessary changes.

Life rewards you when you are true to yourself. A new self emerges to replace the old one. And life will never be the same. ◆

CHAPTER 2
AMERICA'S HEALTH TODAY

The best doctor gives the least medicine.
—Benjamin Franklin

America's health is suffering as a whole. This deterioration goes far beyond a broken health care system. We're addicted to pain pills, sleeping pills, anti-inflammatories and antidepressants. We're sicker than ever. The World Health Organization ranks the United States' health care system as number 37 out of 191 countries.

Despite the fact that Americans spend the most money per year on health care, we're not healthier or living longer than other countries. Of the health areas studied, Americans ranked worse than other countries in nine categories including drug abuse, heart disease, obesity, diabetes, and lung disease.

Americans spend over $360 billion a year filling prescriptions. Harvard University's Dr. John Abramson said, "Costs will keep skyrocketing. About $700 billion is wasted every year in the United States on medications and treatments that are unnecessary or harmful" (Congressional Budget Office).

Without a doubt, a great percentage of the nation's take-home pay goes toward stocking the medicine cabinet. Consumers today spend more each year on drugs than on shoes, furniture, and reading material combined. But we're not getting healthier from drug consumption, rather we're getting sicker.

More than a quarter of American kids and teens take medication on a regular basis, according to Medco Health Solutions, Inc., the biggest U.S. pharmacy-benefit manager. Many medications kids take on a regular basis are well-known, including treatments for asthma and attention deficit disorder. But children and teens take a variety of other medications once considered only for adults, from cholesterol-lowering statins to diabetes pills, antidepressants, sleep drugs, drugs to focus better and antipsychotics. This is disturbing, and the long-term effects of drugs in children are rarely understood.

Prescription drugs and over-the-counter drugs are usually intended to address one specific health issue. But the side effects from these drugs often result in more health problems. There is a perception that drugs prescribed by our medical doctors are, for the most part, generally safe and that the benefits far outweigh the risks. However, research by the Florida Medical Examiners Commission indicates *prescription drugs kill more Americans each year than illegal drugs.* This fact alone should motivate us to get to the root cause of our problems and not mask symptoms with prescription and over-the-counter drugs.

Let's look at statistics for the diseases that plague the nation.

Diabetes

More than 100 million U.S. adults are now living with diabetes or prediabetes, according to the Centers for Disease Control and Prevention (CDC 2017). Diabetes is one of the most common diseases in school-aged children. The American Diabetes Association (ADA) estimates the total costs of diagnosed diabetes have risen to $245 billion. This figure represents a 41% increase over a five-year period.

Are We Winning the War on Diabetes?

Diabetes is becoming more common in the United States. The number of Americans with diagnosed diabetes has more than tripled (from 5.6 million to 20.9 million) in the past five years. In spite of over $12 billion being spent annually on finding a cure for diabetes, the cost of treating diabetes continues to rise.

The American Diabetes Association constantly requests donations to support diabetic research that they say will hopefully lead to a cure. After so many years of spending billions annually in search of a cure, a cure for diabetes has not as yet been found.

Diabesity

The combination of diabetes and obesity, now termed "diabesity" by Dr. Mark Hyman, author of *The Blood Sugar Solution*. Diabesity describes the spectrum of metabolic imbalance and disease that ranges from mild blood-sugar imbalance to insulin resistance to full-blown diabetes. According to Dr. Hyman "One in two Americans is suffering from diabesity, and most of them don't even know it. Diabesity can be prevented, treated and reversed."

Arthritis

About 54.4 million adults are clinically diagnosed with arthritis, and another 23.7 million have activity limitation attributable to arthritis. These estimates do not include the average person walking around with undiagnosed aches and pains. As the population ages, clinically diagnosed arthritis is expected to increase and affect an estimated 67 million adults in the United States by 2030.

Obesity

Obesity has become a national health crisis in the U.S. Overall, 40% of American adults are obese. Childhood obesity is a national epidemic. Nearly 1 in 3 children (ages 2-19) in the United States is overweight or obese, putting them at risk for serious health problems.

America.org states that obesity is a leading cause of preventable death in the United States. These statistics worry experts about whether health care costs will increase even further if nothing brings the epidemic under control. "If nothing is done about obesity, it's going to hinder efforts for health care cost containment," says Justin Trogdon, a research economist with RTI International.

Extra weight may indeed take a major toll on health. Obesity increases the risks of type 2 diabetes, heart disease, stroke, many types of cancer, sleep apnea, and other debilitating and chronic illnesses. These effects indicate why obesity contributes enormously to increased health care spending during the past twenty years.

Metabolic Syndrome ("Syndrome X")

Researchers at U.S. Reuters estimated that as many as 68 million Americans exhibit a cluster of medical conditions ("Metabolic Syndrome" or "Syndrome X") characterized by:

1. Insulin resistance and the presence of obesity
2. Excessive abdominal fat
3. High blood sugar and triglycerides
4. High blood pressure (hypertension)
5. High cholesterol

Syndrome X is a direct result of consuming overly processed, fake foods that are accepted as normal in our American way of life. Unfortunately, our lifestyle has created our Western diseases and our dependency on prescription and over-the-counter drugs to combat Syndrome X.

Cancer

Cancer remains one of our most urgent health concerns and the disease many fear most. During recent decades, the incidence of cancer has escalated to epidemic proportions, now striking nearly one in two men (44%) and more than one in three women (39%). As admitted by recent National Cancer Institute and American Cancer Society estimates, the number of cancer cases may further increase due to the growth and aging of the population, which is estimated to dramatically double by 2050.

Heart Disease

Nearly one in three Americans live with some form of heart disease, including high blood pressure, cardiovascular disease, stroke, angina (chest pain), heart attack, and congenital heart defects. It may be America's number one killer, but people aren't scared enough of heart disease, said a top U.S. research cardiologist.

"We've done a good job of advertising to people that we're doing better with heart disease, so people tend to feel good about it," said Dr. Robert Califf, vice-chancellor for clinical research at Duke

University Medical Center. "We have bypass surgery and stents and drugs that work; the [mortality] rates are declining."

"It's sort of accepted as part of the background noise, even though it's far and away the most likely reason that you or I will die," Califf said. "We're just on the front end of the baby boomer epidemic, where the projections on the amount of cardiovascular disease are climbing steadily over the next ten years."

"We're delaying the disease, but we're not preventing it," said Dr. Steven Nissen, president of the American College of Cardiology and chairman of cardiovascular medicine at the Cleveland Clinic in Ohio.

In Conclusion

As statistics continue to rise in all of these chronic health categories, our hope is that Americans wake up to the harsh reality of our nation's declining health and become more motivated to resolve health issues at a deeper level.

CHAPTER 3
REASONS FOR OUR
DECLINING HEALTH

The greatest wealth is health.

Listed below are the obvious (and not so obvious) contributors of chronic disease plaguing Americans today.

1. **Soil Depletion.** Let's start with the basics. Years ago, food harvested from the fields was covered with diverse micro-organisms. Now much of our soil is sterile, resulting in soil depletion. Shortly after World War II, before chemical farming was introduced, all foods were organic: grown without pesticides, herbicides, chemical fertilizers, hormones, or irradiation to prevent spoilage. Foods were unrefined, whole, or minimally processed. Today, much of the world's soils and foods are depleted of minerals and other nutrients. This soil imbalance contributes to the imbalance of bacteria in our gut.

Nowadays our food, whether vegetable or animal, is not only deficient in nutrients but also contaminated with pollutants and farm chemicals. Massive refining of foods through modern manufacturing deeply affects the life-giving nutritional content of food. This change makes maintaining good health more difficult. Research shows that organic produce is more nutrient dense because the soil itself has more minerals and nutrients. A long-term study conducted at the University of California, Davis found higher levels of antioxidants in organic produce. For example, organic tomatoes contained 79% and 97% higher levels of quercetin and kaempferol, respectively. Organic red wines contain higher levels of resveratrol, polyphenols, and other antioxidants.

2. **Hormones and Antibiotics**. These additives are injected into cows, chickens, turkeys, lambs, pigs, and even fish to further insult our food supply. We ingest these chemicals without much thought, but let's not be fooled into believing they're good for us. The biotech mogul Monsanto, responsible for engineering the hormone rBST and the herbicide Roundup, is also the biggest company manufacturing genetically modified food. It is suspected that these synthetic hormones, pesticides, and antibiotics may have an ill effect on our bodies.

3. **Genetically Modified Organism (GMO)**. Non-GMO food sounds like something you wouldn't want, but non-GMO means that the plant is not injected with foreign genes, strange viruses, or bacteria in a laboratory. Non-GMO means real food that exists in nature. The public remains largely unaware about these practices that threaten our health and the safety of our food. The government puts the burden of labeling on the organic farmer. In lab animals, GMOs are linked to thousands of toxic and allergic reactions and damage virtually every organ and system studied. The government admits it does not regulate this alteration of food. Biotech companies have been left in charge of determining whether their foods are safe for human consumption, but these companies are boosting their profits while claiming to feed the world. We believe GMO products—namely, corn, potatoes, canola oil, soy, and cotton—should be avoided whenever possible.

The American Academy of Environmental Medicine links GMO foods with adverse health effects, and the President's Cancer Panel Report on Environmental Cancer Risk Factors recommends that Americans avoid GMO foods due to the increase of cancer risk.

4. **Modern (Hybridized) Wheat**. In the 1970s, a well-meaning geneticist created a hybridized strain of high-yield dwarf wheat. By 1985, all wheat products were made from this altered dwarf strain, which now comprises 99% of all wheat grown worldwide. This wheat converts to blood sugar more easily than almost all other food carbohydrates, which means this grain raises blood sugar higher than nearly all other foods, including table sugar. The reaction contributes

to diabetes, weight gain, food allergies and sensitivities, irritable bowel syndrome, and many other conditions.

5. **Overconsumption of Sugar, High Fructose Corn Syrup (HFCS), and Artificial Sugar.** The average person consumes 100-140 pounds of sugar annually. Our bodies were never meant to consume so much sugar, and we were never meant to consume artificial sugar! Sugar suppresses the immune system by 50% within fifteen minutes of ingesting. Sugar, artificial sugar, and synthetic chemicals form acid inside the body. What loves acid and sugar? Toxins, fungus, bacteria, mold, yeast, and cancer cells.

We'll be taking a closer look at sugar in the chapter, "Sugar and Its Many Disguises."

6. **Trans Fats/Hydrogenated Oils.** Hydrogenation is how muffins manufactured on the East Coast are still soft on the West Coast a week later. Where do you find these types of oils? In margarine, shortenings, baked goods, chocolate, ice cream, potato chips, salad dressing, and nondairy creamers.

Hydrogenation changes an unsaturated, liquid oil into a saturated, more solid fat. This physical change not only alters the nutritional value of the oil, but it actually promotes inflammation in our bodies, contributing to disease.

7. **Stress.** Between 60% and 70% of people end up at a doctor's office or the hospital for stress-related conditions. Overworking, overeating, or substance dependency prevent us from living the full potential of our lives.

Research in the new field of epigenetics is showing this very clearly. It's the interaction of our genes and our environment, which includes lifestyle choices, how we behave, how and what we habitually think, and whether or not we practice mindfulness that determines our susceptibility to various diseases.

We have many healthy options and resources for facing our stressors; we need to make this a priority.

8. **Processed Food.** We have drifted away, both individually and as a nation, from wholesome, real, live, natural, nourishing, chemical-

free, single-ingredient foods. What we eat affects our minds as well as our bodies and is intricately connected to our outlook, mood, energy, and spirit. Giving up processed food may seem like a drastic change, but when you realize how much better you feel and how far the benefits extend, the choices get easier. We may not control what we are exposed to environmentally, but we do control what goes into our bodies. What we put into or minds as well as our bodies is essential to whole body wellness.

Time to Wake Up

Our health challenges took us down a path we might otherwise not have considered and provided an opportunity to become more conscious, awake human beings. Throughout this book, stories are shared about personal wake-up calls intended to provide hope and inspiration.

Here are words of wisdom from a Swiss-American teenager.

Natural Medicine Can Do Wonders—Sarah C.

I spent the first ten years of my life in Switzerland, where natural medicine is already an important part of the medical system. When it comes to health and wellness, the Swiss are ranked number one.

Thanks to their health system, the Swiss have universal coverage and the healthiest population in the Western Hemisphere.

So when I got sick, natural medicine wasn't a new concept to me or my family since it was the only kind of medicine I was used to.

When I came to the U.S., many things were different and I was given contrasting perspectives on ways of life. For one thing, it's against the law in Switzerland to market prescription drugs to the general public. This is drastically different in America; most of the advertisements one sees on television and in magazines are for pharmaceutical drugs.

Knowing there are alternatives to pharmaceuticals gave me an advantage when I went to my traditional doctor for help and all she did was suggest painkillers such as Aleve and Tylenol.

I then went to see a naturopathic doctor (N.D.) instead and got the help I needed. She wanted to know my background and about one of the most vital things that Western doctors don't focus on: nutrition. This makes little sense since the large majority of the illnesses these doctors will attempt to treat are caused by a lack of proper nutrition (or the need to eliminate certain foods from one's diet.)

My N.D. connected every past and current problem I had and knew instantly what was wrong with me, and even better, that there was a way to free myself of it.

When people visit a doctor, they normally aren't aware of the type of doctor that they're going to see. The traditionally-trained doctor in the U.S. is trained very differently than a holistic doctor, also known as a natural medicine practitioner or naturopathic doctor.

Many of us trust our doctors completely, so when we are given a pharmaceutical, we take it as we are told without question. However, often it is unnecessary and doesn't fix the underlying problem. It only covers it up and neglects the body as a whole, essentially causing damage to other parts of the body.

Homeopathy, acupuncture, meditation, traditional Chinese medicine and nutritional remedies are all types of alternative medicine that have been used successfully for thousands of years.

Drug-based therapies are known as conventional medicine, which have only come into existence relatively recently.

Logically, it seems we've switched these two.

The therapies that people have used with success for so many years are treated as an alternative even though they should be the standard. Complementary medicine, medicine that I've used to help heal myself, treats the body as a whole rather than so many separate parts.

Natural medicine finds ways to cure supposedly incurable diseases, and an increasing number of people are turning to alternatives for treatment.

Unfortunately, the majority of us are not aware of just how effective natural medicine is.

Our money-driven society has persuaded us that pharmaceuticals are the only "real" medicine, but this experience has taught me to approach things with an open mind. Healing begins with finding the core of the problem. This realization saved me from a life of serious health problems and made me aware of and embrace the rapidly growing field of holistic medicine. ♦

Holistic Approach: Functional and Integrative Medicine

Functional and integrative medicine are complementary approaches to Western medicine. Functional medicine looks at the underlying causes of disease, and patient and practitioner work together from a more patient-centered outlook. By shifting the traditional disease-centered focus of Western medical practice, functional medicine addresses the whole person, not just a set of symptoms.

From our experience, most Western medicine doctors do not account for each individual's unique genetic makeup or factors such as exposure to toxins and lifestyle (diet, thoughts, stress, and exercise). These factors have a direct influence on chronic disease. Doctors who practice functional medicine emphasize the whole person, not merely the symptoms. This approach facilitates prevention through supplements, therapeutic diets, detoxification programs, stress-management techniques, and exercise as well as the use of laboratory testing.

These practitioners spend time with their patients and listen to their stories. They bring the patient into the discovery process and tailor treatments that address the needs of the individual. This method supports unique expressions of health and vitality. This form of medicine asks the questions, "Why? Which system is out of balance?" and offers more than the right drug for a disease.

Integrative medicine combines conventional Western medicine with alternative or complementary treatments, such as herbal medicine, acupuncture, massage, biofeedback, yoga, and stress reduction techniques.

Our philosophy encourages you to take personal responsibility for your health. The age of being a passive patient and placing medical doctors on pedestals is coming to an end.

Hospitals use the terms "wellness," "prevention," and "thrive" in their advertising and marketing campaigns, but in most medical schools there is little if any time spent on understanding preventative measures for chronic, degenerative disease. After all, medical schools and conferences are often supported and sponsored by drug manufacturers who are disinterested in promoting nutritional therapies.

We will most likely always need allopathic doctors to fix broken bones, remove diseased body parts, or for emergency care in the case of accidents. And for these kinds of procedures we are very grateful.

In Conclusion

As integrative, functional and holistic medicine become more mainstream, Americans will find and treat the underlying cause of their disease rather than merely treat their symptoms.

CHAPTER 4
MINDFUL EATING

Your physical condition tomorrow starts with what you're doing for your body and what you're thinking about today. Choose wisely.

Mindfulness is moment-to-moment awareness. Mindfulness is bigger than thought and gives us more freedom in how we react to life. Mindful eating is about paying attention—to our bodies, our thoughts, our food, and our emotions. When we're not paying attention, we get disconnected. When we get disconnected from ourselves, we get into stress and tension. Then we're more prone to disease.

What heals arthritis is often the same approach as what heals diabetes and other conditions. Our philosophy is that mindful eating is the most influential and fundamental thing you can do to have the most positive impact on your health and your life.

When we are practicing mindfulness, we're being present in the moment. When we are present in the moment, we are getting a break from our routine-oriented thoughts. This makes space for a new idea, a new perspective, or a new way of thinking to arise. Practicing mindfulness gives us an opportunity to see ourselves in a new light.

What Is Mindful Eating?

Mindful eating is the first step for reclaiming your health and your life. When you eat mindfully, you are in touch with your food because your mind is not distracted, or at least it is less distracted. When you chew, you really taste your food. When you eat mindfully, you tune into your body and take a moment to sense what your body is wanting and needing.

We hope to elevate your awareness about mindful eating and all those seemingly "small" decisions you make each and every day that affect all aspects of your being.

Mindful eating is a conscious choice to truly nourish your body. It begins with these six steps:

1. **Be more curious about the source of your food.** Begin to question "Where is the food from? Is it organic, raised on a farm, free-range, wild-caught, local?

2. **Select high quality food** such as Non-GMO (non-genetically modified organism)

Chemical-, hormone-, pesticide-, and antibiotic–free. All whole foods are not necessarily high quality. For example, if the corn or potato has been genetically modified, then it's lost some of its wholeness and quality. Is it free of processing, high fructose corn syrup, trans fats, hydrogenated oils, and artificial sugars?

3. **Slow down when eating**

To create a low stress environment.

So that you are fully aware of the present moment.

In order to focus on the taste of the food.

To digest, metabolize, and process food better. Eating fast causes us to eat more because we don't have a chance to feel full and this results in poor digestion.

4. **Pay attention to how food makes you feel**

Keep a notebook handy. Note how you feel after a meal and later that day. Many people have food sensitivities and don't make the connection that their headache came from something they ate and are sensitive to.

5. **Choose consciously**

Mindful eating is about decisions we make every day.

All decisions have impact on our well-being (like what you choose for breakfast).

6. **Take time to be grateful**

Taking a moment to be grateful to the source of our food (from the earth to the farmer to the table) raises the life force of our food, thus raising our own life force energy.

In Conclusion

What we eat and how we eat affects our entire being (emotional, mental, physical, spiritual). When we take time to eat mindfully, our bodies and our spirits soar.

CHAPTER 5
FOODS THAT HEAL

*You don't have to cook fancy or complicated masterpieces, just good
food from fresh ingredients.*
—Julia Child

Since diet is the most controllable factor for preventing and
reversing chronic disease, this chapter is devoted to health and healing
through consuming foods that heal.

We hear it all the time: eat more fruits and vegetables (preferably
organic). The USDA's MyPlate, helps address the growing obesity
problem in the U.S. These guidelines serve as the "cornerstone of
federal nutrition policy and nutrition education activities." MyPlate
recommends making half your plate vegetables and fruit. What makes
plants so healing?

The Power of Greens
Leafy greens are the most beneficial vegetables to incorporate into
your daily routine. However, they are the most absent food group
from the American diet. We recommend increasing your intake of
veggies. Here's why:

Leafy green vegetables are densely-packed with energy and
nutrients and grow upwards toward the sky, absorbing the sun's light
while producing oxygen. Members of the royal green family include
kale, collard greens, Swiss chard, mustard greens, arugula, dandelion
greens, watercress, beet greens, bok choy, cabbage, spinach, and
broccoli.

How do greens benefit our bodies? They are high in calcium,
magnesium, iron, potassium, phosphorous, and zinc, and are a
powerhouse for vitamins A, C, E, and K. They are crammed full of

fiber, folic acid, chlorophyll, and many other micronutrients and phytochemicals.

Phytochemicals are plant chemicals that have protective or disease preventive properties. Most phytochemicals have antioxidant activity and protect our cells against oxidative damage and reduce the risk of certain types of cancer. Some fruits are also high (though not as high as greens) in phytochemicals, such as strawberries, blueberries, cranberries, cherries, goji berries, mangosteen, and acai.

Greens aid in:

- purifying the blood
- helping the liver to detoxify blood
- strengthening the immune system
- improving liver, gall bladder, and kidney function
- fighting depression
- clearing congestion
- improving circulation
- keeping your skin clear

Below are twenty-five super foods which are nutrient-dense foods that have powerful antioxidant properties. Nutrient density refers not only to vitamins and minerals, but also to phytochemicals essential for proper functioning of the immune system, enabling the body's detoxification and cellular repair mechanisms that protect it from chronic diseases. Not surprisingly, leafy greens top the list:

1. collard, mustard, and turnip greens
2. kale
3. watercress
4. bok choy
5. spinach
6. brussels sprouts
7. swiss chard
8. arugula
9. radish

10. cabbage
11. red peppers
12. romaine lettuce
13. broccoli
14. carrot juice
15. tomatoes
16. cauliflower
17. strawberries
18. pomegranate juice
19. blackberries
20. plums
21. raspberries
22. blueberries
23. papaya
24. Brazil nuts
25. oranges

The Power of Juicing

There is a miracle of energy supplied by organic, live plants that comes from nothing else on the planet. After all has been investigated and analyzed, it still can't be fully explained. "Juice therapy" has worked to bring about recovery from illness for many people. A study published in *The American Journal of Medicine* reports that both vegetable and fruit juice may help protect against Alzheimer's disease due to the phytochemical polyphenol. Not only does juicing provide more of these phytochemicals, it also provides the body with more water.

Juicing is an easy way of putting a diversity of flavorful, nutrient-dense beverages into your diet. Fresh fruits and vegetables have powerful, protective effects for the body. Juice from fresh, organic fruits and vegetables is the richest available food source of vitamins, minerals, and enzymes—the stuff of life.

Juicing enables your body to easily assimilate the many valuable nutrients in food. Enzymes in raw foods help break down and absorb all the nutrients, but are destroyed when foods are cooked. The quick and easy digestion of raw foods, made possible by the enzymes, will give you greater energy and health.

Jay Kordich, referred to as the father of juicing, authored the best-selling book *The Juiceman's Power of Juicing.* He is famous for the statement, "All life on earth emanates from the green of the plant."

Dr. Bircher-Benner, a well-known doctor who founded a famous clinic in Switzerland said, "Nothing more therapeutic exists on earth than green juices."

Fruit and veggie juice offers you a concentration of nutrients packed together to nourish your body and enhance your health. So just how much should we be consuming?

Many health experts say seven veggie servings and two fruits per day. Evidence suggests that eating your food raw provides more energy and slows the rate at which you age.

Getting Started

How does one begin increasing his/her intake of raw foods? Begin slowly, and pay attention to how your body feels and responds. You'll need a high-power blender like a Vitamix or similar machine and juice often. This is one way that busy people, such as parents and children, can consume the fruits and vegetables they need to achieve optimal health.

Juicing is made simple by blending fruits and vegetables with about thirty percent ice, water, or other liquids (lemon juice, lime juice, or another extracted juice). Adding a couple strawberries or one-quarter of an apple to your bitter greens is a great way to sweeten the taste and make your green juices more enjoyable.

If a juice fast appeals to you, be sure to pick a time when you know your activity will not be as strenuous as usual. When the time comes to break your fast, be sure to eat lightly and slowly—some whole fruit, perhaps. Do *not* fast if you're diabetic, pregnant, or nursing.

Juicing can increase the release of toxins passing through your system. Some people can only handle a limited amount of juicing, as the toxins going through their system can make them feel achy and worse. In this case, making a smoothie with other ingredients such as nut milks, kefir/yogurt, protein powder, a handful of greens, and a half banana or apple can provide a healthy smoothie without any ill effects. Experiment with what feels best for your body.

Why Eat Organic?

According to Andrew Weil, MD, the three most important reasons to choose organic foods are because they are:

1) Safer (since you are not consuming pesticides)

2) Better for the environment

3) More nutritious

To get the most health benefits from eating fruits and vegetables, organic or "pesticide free" is your best choice.

Originally, all foods were "organic," meaning they were grown and prepared without pesticides, herbicides, chemical fertilizers, hormones, or irradiation to prevent spoilage, etc. Foods were unrefined, whole, or at most, minimally processed. Since World War II and the advent of chemical farming and food processing, the soils and foods of much of the world have been depleted of minerals and other nutrients.

Is avoiding pesticides on fruits and vegetables really worth the extra cost? Pesticides have been linked to birth defects and shown to cause cancer, as well as liver, kidney, and blood diseases. As pesticides get lodged in our tissues, our immune systems become weakened, allowing other carcinogens and pathogens to affect our health. Without a doubt, pesticides are chemicals used to prevent, destroy, or repel pests. Many experts, such as biology professor David Ehrenfeld, MD, author of *Becoming Good Ancestors: How We Balance Nature, Community, and Technology*, caution that pesticides have been linked to various health problems.

If you have kids, you should be especially concerned. Children eat two to four times more produce than adults, relative to their body weight, which increases their pesticide exposure, according to Natalie Geary, MD, a New York City pediatrician. "Unfortunately, when exposure occurs as their organs and bones are still growing, it can affect normal development."

Are there health benefits to eating organic produce? The answer is yes. Organic produce has higher antioxidant levels than conventional produce according to a 2014 study at Washington State University's Center for Sustaining Agriculture and Natural Resources. Organic crops and crop-based foods contain as much as 60% more antioxidants than conventional crops. The significance of this is comparable to eating an additional one to two extra fruit or vegetable servings a day. Antioxidants have been linked to a lower risk of cancer and other diseases.

The modern denaturing of foods through refining and chemical treatment deeply affects the life force, making it difficult to foster equilibrium and health. Our food these days, whether of vegetable or animal origin, is not only deficient in antioxidants but also full of pollutants and farm chemicals.

Organic certification is a promise to consumers that products have been grown and handled according to strict procedures without persistent toxic chemical inputs.

10 Reasons to Shop for and Eat Organic Foods

1. **Keep chemicals off your plate.** Pesticides are poisons designed to kill living organisms, and can also be harmful to humans. Many Environmental Protection Agency (EPA)-approved pesticides were registered long before extensive research linked these chemicals to cancer and other diseases.

2. **Flavor and Nourishment.** Organic farming starts with the nourishment of the soil, thereby producing nourished and nourishing plants. Well-balanced soil produces strong, healthy plants, which in turn produces strong, healthy bodies.

3. **Prevent soil erosion.** Three billion tons of topsoil are eroded from crop lands in the U.S. each year, much of it due to pesticide use, which often ignores the health of the soil.

4. **Protect water quality.** The EPA estimates that pesticides pollute the primary source of drinking water for more than half the U.S. population. hear

5. **Organic farmers work in harmony with nature and promote biodiversity.** Organic agricultural promotes the balance of a healthy ecosystem. Planting large plots of land with the same crop year after year triples farm production, but the lack of natural diversity of plant life negatively affects soil quality. Organic farming promotes biodiversity and healthier soil while most conventional farming does not.

6. **Save energy.** More energy is now used to produce synthetic fertilizers for non-organic farming than to till, cultivate, and harvest all the crops in the U.S.

7. **Help small farmers.** Although more and more large-scale farms are making the conversion to organic practices, most organic farms are small, independently-owned and family-operated farms. Organic agriculture can be a lifeline for small farms because it offers an alternative market where sellers can command fair prices for crops.

8. **Support a true economy.** Organic foods might seem expensive; however, your tax dollars pay for hazardous waste cleanup and environmental damage caused by conventional farming.

9. **Protect future generations.** Organic foods are a healthy, wholesome, safe choice for your family. Children receive four times more exposure than adults to cancer-causing pesticides in foods.

10. **Organic agriculture.** One way to prevent more chemicals from getting into the air, earth, and water that sustain us is organic agriculture. Organic foods do not contain genetically modified organisms (GMOs). Learn more about GMOs below.

Organic Standards

Now, more than ever, we need health regulations that protect children and adults from chemicals that can harm them. Keeping the USDA organic seal pure requires constant vigilance. When we demand organic, we are demanding poison-free food. We are demanding soil that is free to do its job and seeds that are free from toxins.

Food Tips

1. Eat more raw, organic vegetables and fruits as a way to enjoy optimal health and abundant energy.

2. Juicing in a high-power blender is a great way for busy people, parents, and kids to increase consumption of vegetables and fruits.

3. Because of the potential health risks associated with GMO, choose organic or foods that are labeled "Non-GMO." We will discuss this more at length in the next chapter.

4. Consume organic beans and lentils as part of an overall healthy diet (provided you are not an IBS/IBD sufferer).

5. If you drink coffee, make sure it's freshly ground and organic. Enjoy in moderation to reap its many health benefits.

Easy Way to Create a Healthy Meal

Draw an imaginary line down the middle of your plate.

- Fill half of your plate with non-starchy vegetables (salad, spinach, broccoli, asparagus, kale, green beans) using a healthy fat such as olive oil.

- Divide the other side of your plate in half and fill one quarter section with healthy protein such as lean meat or fish.

- Fill the last quarter section with whole grains such as brown rice, quinoa, or a starchy vegetable such as carrots, peas, potatoes, or beans.

In Conclusion

Organic vegetables and fruits are the most healing foods for maintaining good health. It's important to choose organic. While it may cost a bit more, one must consider that these extra costs could be offset by fewer trips to the doctor or paying less on one's medical bills.

CHAPTER 6
GMOS AND ORGANIC FOODS

When it comes to owning the seed for collecting royalties, the GMO companies say, "It's mine." But when it comes to contamination, cross-pollination, and health problems, the response is "We're not liable."
—Dr. Vandana Shiva

The term genetically modified organism (GMO) is known as genetically modified food and refers to crop plants that have been modified in a laboratory to enhance desired traits, such as resistance to herbicides. This type of farming is referred to as "chemical farming." Experts say this science, like any other, has no guarantees.

Now let's take a look at what chemical farming proponents say about how farmers and ranchers are improving with the use of genetically modified seeds in America.

While higher productivity and trade opportunity are valid points, most developed nations do not consider GMOs to be safe. In more than sixty countries around the world, including Australia, Japan, and all of the countries in the European Union, there are significant restrictions or outright bans on the production and sale of GMOs. In the U.S., the government has approved GMOs based on studies conducted by the same corporations that profit from their sale.

Risks Include
- Introducing allergens and toxins to food
- Accidental contamination between genetically modified and non-genetically modified foods
- Antibiotic resistance
- Adversely changing the nutrient content of a crop
- Creation of "super" weeds and other environmental risks

Benefits Include

- Increased pest and disease resistance
- Drought tolerance
- Increased food supply

Here is a list of the eight most common GMO foods so that you can become more aware while grocery shopping.

1. **Soy.** Up to 93% of soybeans in the market have been genetically modified to be naturally resistant to an herbicide called Roundup.

2. **Corn.** 90% of the U.S. farms grow GMO corn. Most of this corn is going to be used for human consumption.

3. **Canola oil.** Canola oil is derived from rapeseed oil. It is considered one of the most chemically altered oils sold in the U.S.

4. **Cotton.** 90% of U.S. cotton has been genetically modified to increase yield and resistance to disease. Most concern relates to cotton oil.

5. **Sugar.** 54% of sugar is genetically modified. Like corn, these sugar beets are modified to resist Roundup.

6. **Aspartame.** Aspartame is a popular artificial sweetener used instead of sugar. Aspartame is manufactured from genetically modified bacteria.

7. **Zucchini and Yellow Squash.** Genetically modified zucchini contains a toxic protein that helps make it more resistant to insects. Some of the insecticide makes its way into our bodies rather than being broken down and excreted.

8. **Papaya.** Genetically modified papaya trees have been grown in Hawaii since 1999. These papayas are sold in the United States and Canada for human consumption.

These are just eight of the most prevalent GMO foods found in the supermarket.

GMO Labeling

The U.S. government has put the burden of labeling on the organic farmer (the USDA Organic label), not the biotech companies like Monsanto. USDA Organic means that the product has undergone rigorous testing and has not been genetically altered or modified. Government subsidizes and gives tax breaks and easy regulations for chemical farming. However, polls consistently show that a significant majority of Americans would like to be able to tell if the food they're purchasing contains GMOs. A CBS news poll found that 87% of consumers wanted GMOs labeled. If you would like to have GMO foods labeled, watch for legislation on this issue, vote, and let your voice be heard.

While grains tend to have lower pesticide residues than produce, organic versions may have more fiber and higher levels of nutrients because they're less processed.

Below is a list of the best and worst non-organic foods according to their pesticide load. If an item you buy often is on the Dirty Dozen list, get in the habit of buying the organic (cleanest) version of that item.

Dirty Dozen	Cleanest Dozen
peaches	onions
apples	avocados
sweet bell peppers	sweet corn (frozen)
celery	pineapples
nectarines	mangoes
strawberries	sweet peas (frozen)
cherries	asparagus
lettuce	kiwi
grapes	bananas
pears	cabbage
spinach	broccoli
potatoes	eggplant

Organizations Supporting Organic & Non-GMO

Organizations such as the Organic Consumers Association (OCA) and the Non-GMO Project have been created to support awareness about GMOs and reasons to go organic when possible. The Non-GMO Project is a nonprofit organization created by leaders representing all sectors of the organic and natural products market in the U.S. and Canada. Its purpose is to offer consumers a consistent non-GMO choice for organic and natural products that are produced without genetic engineering.

The OCA promotes organic food and sustainable agriculture. Increasingly, Americans are taking matters into their own hands and choosing to opt out of the GMO experiment.

Visit Non-GMO Project's website at www.nongmoproject.org for a list of products and brands and visit the Organic Consumers Association at www.organicconsumers.org to learn how you can become more involved.

In Conclusion

Foods labeled "USDA Organic" have long been the gold standard for health and sustainability. Scientists and consumer and environmental groups have cited many health and environmental risks with foods containing GMOs. A smart start is to resist the Dirty Dozen. When you buy organic you are supporting farmers who are committed to the highest food standards. And it's better for you, the environment, and your family.

CHAPTER 7
BEANS, BEANS

Beans or legumes stabilize blood sugar, blunt the desire for sweets,
and prevent mid-afternoon cravings.
—Joel Fuhrman

Beans are a naturally nutritious food and the U.S. Dietary Guidelines recommend we triple our current intake from one to three cups per week. The term legumes includes beans, peas and lentils.

There are many factors that make beans good for us, and they are the best sources of lean vegetarian protein. Although beans have many positive attributes, there is also a downside to eating beans.

Let's First Take a Look at the Positive Attributes of Beans

These heart-healthy nutrients help lower blood pressure and can reduce your risk of coronary artery disease, diabetes, and osteoporosis. Many studies suggest that the folate in beans can improve mood and memory, while magnesium prevents migraine headaches and works with potassium to normalize blood pressure.

Soluble fiber, in particular, keeps you feeling fuller for longer, so it's a good tool for weight loss. One cup of cooked beans provides about twelve grams of fiber—nearly half the recommended daily dose of twenty-one to twenty-five grams per day for adult women (thirty to thirty-eight grams for adult men).

Some legumes contain additional nutrients, such as zinc or vitamin B6. Zinc is a mineral that contributes to tissue growth and repair; it helps keep your skin and hair healthy. This mineral is also found in the retina of the eye, where it helps fend off macular degeneration. Vitamin B6 protects against age-related memory decline and also maintains healthy hair.

Beans are also high in antioxidants, a class of phytochemicals that incapacitate cell-damaging free radicals in the body. Free radicals have been implicated in everything from cancer and aging to neurodegenerative diseases like Parkinson's and Alzheimer's.

Common varieties of beans include black beans, kidney beans, lima beans, navy beans, pinto beans, white beans, soybeans (edamame), and garbanzo beans (chickpeas).

Black beans pack in a good amount of protein, soluble fiber, folate, iron, potassium, and other heart-healthy nutrients. They are also rich in magnesium, so they can help ward off migraine headaches.

In addition to their other heart-healthy nutrients, kidney beans contain vitamin C, an antioxidant that is responsible for the production of collagen, a component of cartilage. This vitamin helps prevent and manage arthritis and contributes to healthy skin and hair. Vitamin C has also been shown to help reduce the risk and progression of macular degeneration. Kidney beans also contain niacin, a B vitamin that may prevent cataracts. And like black beans, they are rich in magnesium, so they may have additional health benefits for people who suffer from migraines.

Garbanzo beans (chickpeas) and lima beans are high in zinc. Besides zinc, garbanzo beans contain migraine-fighting magnesium, vitamin B6, and they're exceptionally high in folate.

White beans are a good nondairy source of calcium, so they can help maintain strong bones and fight PMS symptoms. They're also rich in quercetin, an anti-inflammatory antioxidant that helps prevent and manage arthritis and guard against memory loss.

Lentils, split peas, black-eyed peas, and most other legumes are high in soluble fiber, lean protein, folate, magnesium, potassium, and zinc. Lentils also contain vitamin B6, and they're especially high in iron and folate.

The bottom line? Beans can be seen as pretty much the perfect food for many people but not for all and here's why.

The Downside of Beans

Although beans contain the most protein of plant foods, eating meat, dairy, fish and eggs will bring more protein into your diet

Beans contain lectins that can cause problems for many people. One major concern is that lectins can trigger inflammation in the body. C-reactive protein (CRP) is used as a marker of inflammation and is one example of the many lectins you have circulating in your body. People struggling with inflammatory or autoimmune disease, pre-diabetes or diabetes conditions may need to be particularly careful with lectins. Overgrowth of bacteria can occur in the gut and can result in gas and inflammation.

Some people with irritable bowel syndrome (IBS) are especially sensitive to the insoluble fiber in legumes. Dr. Mark Hyman in his book *Food, What the Heck Should I Eat,* says IBS is often caused by overgrowth of bad bugs in the small intestine or colon.

He states, "Humans don't produce gas. Bugs eating your food and fermenting it create it. And those bugs go crazy for the starch in beans." So if you suffer from IBS and find legumes problematic, you'll want to limit them in your diet."

Among the most lectin containing foods are wheat, beans, soy and other legumes, grains, and in the nightshade family such as tomatoes, peppers, eggplant, and potatoes (not yams). Grains, cereal, dairy, and legumes (especially peanut and soybean) lectins are most commonly associated with reports of digestive complaints. Legumes and seafood are the most abundant sources of lectins in most diets.

The good news is that fermenting, sprouting and cooking will decrease lectins and free up the good nutrients. Using a pressure cooker is best for reducing lectins.

Preparing and Cooking Dried Beans

Begin by washing beans and discarding any that are discolored or badly formed. Check for debris in the package such as small rocks or twigs and discard them. Beans cook quicker and their digestibility benefits increase if you soak them in water to cover by about three inches for eight hours or overnight. Afterward, discard the soak water and cook the beans in fresh water.

There are many types of beans available. The following chart describes nine of the most common varieties of beans available in U.S. supermarkets. The cooking time refers to the time needed to cook dry beans.

Bean Chart

Beans	Description	Cooking Time
Black	**Black Beans** are medium-sized, oval-shaped beans with matte black skin. They are also called turtle beans. They are sweet tasting with a soft texture. Popular beans in Central American, South American, and Caribbean cuisine.	60-90 minutes
Cranberry	**Cranberry Beans** are medium-sized, oval-shaped beans with mottled tan–and–red skin. They are also known as Roman beans. Cranberry beans are known for their creamy texture with a flavor similar to chestnuts. The red specks disappear when these beans are cooked. Cranberry beans are a favorite in northern Italy and Spain.	45-60 minutes

Great Northern	**Great Northern Beans** are medium-sized, oval-shaped beans with thin white skin. They have a delicate flavor. Great Northern beans are very popular in France for making a white bean casserole and in the Mediterranean where many beans of a similar appearance are cultivated.	45-60 minutes
Dark Red Kidney	**Dark Red Kidney Beans** are large, kidney-shaped beans with a deep, glossy red skin. They have a firm texture, and they hold up well in soups or other dishes that cook for a long time. Dark red kidney beans are used in soups, cold bean salads, and chili. Both dark and red kidney beans are used to make Louisiana Red Beans & Rice.	90-120 minutes
Light Red Kidney	**Light Red Kidney Beans** are large, kidney-shaped beans with light red/pink glossy skin. They have a firm texture, and they hold up well in soups or other dishes that cook for a long time. Light Red Kidney beans are popular in the Caribbean region, Portugal and Spain. Both dark and red kidney beans are used to make Louisiana Red Beans & Rice.	90-120 minutes

Navy	**Navy Beans** are small, oval-shaped beans with white skin. They have a delicate flavor. These are the beans used for the famous Boston Baked Beans. These white beans were named navy beans because of their inclusion in the U.S. naval diet during the second half of the nineteenth century.	90-120 minutes
Pink	**Pink Beans** are small, oval-shaped beans with a pale, pink skin. Pink beans are very popular in Caribbean countries. They are used to make Caribbean Pink Beans, a dish made with no added fat and flavored with sofrito, a mixture of tomatoes, bell peppers, onions, and garlic.	60 minutes
Pinto	**Pinto Beans** are medium-sized, oval-shaped beans with mottled beige–and–brown skin. Like cranberry beans, pinto beans lose their mottled appearance when cooked. Pinto beans are the most widely produced bean in the United States and one of the most popular in the Americas. Pinto beans are used to make Mexican refried beans.	90-120 minutes

 Small Red	**Small Red Beans** are small, oval-shaped beans with red skin. They have a more delicate flavor and softer texture compared to kidney beans. Small red beans are particularly popular in the Caribbean region, where they normally are eaten with rice.	60-90 minutes

In Conclusion

Beans can be a good source of lean vegetarian protein and are rich in vitamins, minerals, and fiber. These heart-healthy nutrients can improve mood, help lower blood pressure and reduce your risk of coronary artery disease, diabetes, and osteoporosis.

CHAPTER 8
OUR LOVE AFFAIR WITH
COFFEE AND CHOCOLATE

I'll read my books and I'll drink coffee and I'll listen to music, and
I'll bolt the door.
—J.D. Salinger

People from all over the world drink and love their coffee. Nowadays, with over 400 billion cups consumed every year, coffee is the world's most popular drink. What makes coffee so special?

Some love the taste, while others the caffeinated kick-start that gets them going, especially in the morning. Though not a big fan of coffee himself, Dr. Mehmet Oz understands well why people drink it. "In this fast-paced, hectic, pulled-in-all-directions era, we crave more mojo to perform better in our jobs, to be more engaged with our families, and to attack each day with more spunk." Coffee is also a diuretic, which helps keep the digestive system moving. The good news is there are actually even more reasons to drink coffee.

Coffee Pros

1. **Coffee may protect against type 2 diabetes.**

Researchers at UCLA identified plasma levels of the protein sex hormone binding globulin (SHBG). SHBG controls the biological activity of the body's sex hormones (testosterone and estrogen), which play a role in the development of type 2 diabetes.

Harvard School of Public Health (HSPH) gathered data from three studies. The researchers found that the participants whose coffee intake was –two to two and a half cups a day over a four-year period had an 11% lower type 2 diabetes risk over the subsequent four years, compared with people who did not change their intake.

2. Coffee may lower the risk of liver cancer.

Italian researchers found that coffee consumption lowers the risk of liver cancer by about 40%. The lead author of the study, Dr. Carlo La Vecchia, from Milan's Istituto di Ricerche Farmacologiche Mario Negri, said, "Our research confirms past claims that coffee in moderation of two to two and a half cups a day is good for your health and particularly the liver."

3. Coffee may help prevent liver disease.

Regular consumption of coffee is linked to a reduced risk of primary sclerosing cholangitis (PSC), a rare autoimmune disease of the bile ducts in the liver.

In addition, coffee consumption can lower the incidence of cirrhosis of the liver for alcohol drinkers by 22%, according to a study at the Kaiser Permanente Medical Care Program, California, USA.

4. Fresh, organic coffee contains antioxidant bioflavonoids.

Bioflavonoids are potent, free radical scavengers that reduce oxidative stress on the cell and also possess anti-inflammatory properties. "Decaffeinated" tea or coffee loses this benefit in the processing. One cup of brewed black coffee has more of these antioxidants than three oranges, but the coffee must be consumed *fresh* within twenty minutes of being made, as the strength and amount of the bioflavonoids decreases after that time.

5. Coffee may protect the brain

Research has shown that both whole cocoa beans and coffee have remarkable neuroprotective properties. Emerging evidence supports that South American societies who drink freshly ground coffee from whole coffee beans have the lowest rates of Alzheimer's and Parkinson's disease.

Coffee Cons

Drinking coffee has become so addictive that some people can't get through the day without drinking several cups morning, noon, and night. It has even evolved into a social drink, with consumers spending generously on sugar-loaded concoctions from cafes around the globe.

1. Addiction can result in drinking too much coffee. Overconsumption can result in the following:
- fluid loss in your body
- rheumatoid arthritis
- adrenal fatigue
- stroke
- damaged blood vessels
- insomnia
- anxiety symptoms
- depleted calcium and iron levels in women

2. **Pesticides.** Most coffee produced today is heavily contaminated with pesticides. It's actually one of the most heavily sprayed crops. To ensure compliance with organic industry standards, look for the USDA 100% Organic seal. If you have trouble finding organic coffee in your local grocery store, check online as there are many organic coffees available.

3. **Stale Coffee.** Most coffee is packed from ground beans that cannot survive even a week before getting stale. This is because the rate of rancidity increases dramatically once you grind the beans. Much of the bagged coffee you find in the grocery store is an already degraded product with rancid oils inside. All that will give you is the caffeine. It won't provide you with healthful nutritional co-factors. So grind the coffee beans of your choice fresh, making sure they are organic and pesticide free.

4. **Coffee is acid–forming**. When your body becomes too acidic, due to an overly acid–forming diet, you set yourself up for a total metabolic shutdown. Over–acidification of your body wastes your muscle and bone tissues, and as the level of acid rises, cellular congestion occurs along with increased vulnerability to degenerative disease.

People with a compromised immune system may do best avoiding coffee altogether.

If you enjoy drinking coffee, do so in moderation. Coffee can be dehydrating, so drink plenty of clean, filtered water throughout the day.

Our Other Love Affair...Chocolate

All you need is love but a little chocolate
now and then doesn't hurt.
—Charles M. Schulz

Nothing says "I love you" better than a box of chocolates. (Between roses and chocolate, there may be some debate.) In today's culture, chocolate is often given as a gift for occasions such as Valentine's Day, Easter, birthdays and Christmas. Many of us are likely to consume a little chocolate every day for its mood–and–energy–boosting effects. The portability and availability of chocolate makes it the perfect pleasure to enjoy anytime, anywhere.

The most nutrient-dense type of chocolate is dark, organic, low sugar, and raw. Raw organic cacao powder is a super food that's super delicious.

With over 300 identifiable chemical compounds, cacao is one of the most complex and pleasurably satisfying foods on the planet. In its raw form, cacao contains anandamide (a euphoric substance), arginine (a natural aphrodisiac), neurotransmitters that stimulate and balance brain activity, tryptophan (an anti-depressant), antioxidants, and other beneficial compounds known to have rejuvenating and anti-aging elements.

Cacao is high in magnesium, which is essential for building strong bones, lowering blood pressure, and helping the heart to pump blood efficiently. In fact, desire for chocolate during the female menstrual cycle may be related to cravings for magnesium, a mineral with calming qualities. Cacao is also a good source of the beauty mineral sulfur, which is responsible for healthy skin, nails, and hair.

There are dark chocolate bars sweetened with Stevia. For example, Lily's Sweets produces "Lily's Dark Chocolate," a brand of natural dark chocolate that incorporates Stevia, in place of sugar (more about Stevia in the Sugar chapter).

Another dark chocolate bar is "Simply Lite." It's sweetened with Maltitol, a sugar alcohol that's not our top choice because it can produce gas in some people.

As discussed in the Artificial Sugars and Healthy Alternatives chapter, our top choices for healthy sugar alternatives are Stevia and Xylitol.

In Conclusion

Coffee in moderation of 2 to 2 1/2 cups a day is good for your health and particularly the liver. However, people with a compromised immune system may do best avoiding coffee altogether.

Cacao contains compounds essential for building strong bones, lowering blood pressure, and helping the heart to pump blood efficiently. Enjoy both in moderation for good health.

CHAPTER 9
A STORY THAT SUPPORTS
HOW FOOD HEALS

Don't eat anything your great-great grandmother
wouldn't recognize as food.
—Michael Pollan

Below is a powerful story that supports the "foods heal" philosophy. The story illustrates how incorporating healthy food changed an entire school.

How Healthy Food Changed an Entire School

Appleton Central Alternative Charter High School (ACA) opened its doors in February of 1996 to give individualized attention to students struggling in conventional schools. Because the school struggled with discipline and weapons violations, a police officer was hired to be on staff. According to Greg Bretthauer, who turned down the job of dean of students at ACA, the students were "rude, obnoxious, and ill-mannered."

Teachers commented that students displayed a lack of concentration and often interrupted their teachers and peers, listened poorly, were off task, did not follow directions, lost their tempers, used profane language, and made inappropriate comments.

In 1997, Natural Ovens of Manitowoc, WI initiated a five-year project to bring healthy food into area schools. The goal was to show that fresh, healthy food could make a real difference in student behavior, learning, and health. Prior to the wellness program, the only food and beverages available were vended items including sodas, candy bars, chips, and other snack foods. Students ate from the vending machines throughout the day.

On a Monday morning, students arrived at ACA to find all soda and candy machines gone. Natural Ovens served the students a healthy breakfast and a fresh, well-balanced lunch, including bottled water.

Teacher Mary Bruyette said that she saw changes "overnight." She noticed a considerable decrease in impulsive behaviors, fidgeting, and use of foul language. Mary believes, "If you've been guzzling Mountain Dew and eating chips and you're flying all over the place, I don't think you're going to pick up a whole lot in class." She reports that the students are now calm and well behaved. "I don't have to deal with the daily discipline issues; that just isn't an issue here."

Complaints of headaches, stomachaches, and feeling tired lessened. Within a short period of time, negative behavior such as vandalism, drug and weapons violations, dropout and expulsion rates, and suicide attempts were all virtually nonexistent. There was a calmness and purposefulness that set these teens apart from others.

In the cafeteria, there was no smell of grease. Burgers, fries, and burritos were replaced with salads, and meats were prepared with old-fashioned recipes and whole grain breads. Fresh fruits and vegetables were offered and the students drank water.

In addition to introducing the Nutrition and Wellness Program, other changes included:

1) integrating character development into the students' course work,
2) playing "relaxation music" softly throughout the school,
3) teachers eating with the students,
4) increasing students' physical activity, and
5) students went from often eating nothing in the morning to eating breakfast.

Today at ACA, grades are up, truancy is no longer a problem, arguments are rare, and teachers are able to spend their time teaching.

Greg Bretthauer became the dean of students in an atmosphere that is vastly different from what he saw in 1997.

Students have learned that healthier food keeps them focused and happier. Dr. Scullen (the doctor in charge of the study) had expected that the healthy diet would improve behavior, but he was pleasantly surprised that it had such an impact on academic performance.

Once teens made the connection between food, behavior, and learning, they enjoyed the benefits. One ACA student said, "I really like the food. It tastes good, it's hot, and it's fresh."

One girl commented, "Now that I concentrate, I think it's easier to get along with people 'cause now I'm paying attention to what they have to say and not just worrying about what I have to say to them."

Another student said, "If you're going for a big test you want to eat great."

The on-campus policeman, Dan Tauber, is able to be a role model now, instead of a disciplinarian. In fact, students have become interested in how he eats in order to stay in such good physical shape and have noticed that their athletic abilities have a lot to do with their diet.

"Returning students are now the advocates for the program. The kids encourage each other," according to Mary Bruyette. "They set the example for the new kids. It works great."

"Nutrition for students should be part of the general operating budget," according to Bruyette. "We're concerned about everything else...new band uniforms, the football team, textbooks. Why not be concerned about nutrition? That seems to me the basis in many cases for creating a positive learning environment."

Principal LuAnn Coenen says, "I can't buy the argument that it's too costly for schools to provide good nutrition for their students. I found that one cost will reduce another. I don't have the vandalism, the litter, or the need for high security. We've got to stop using our most precious commodity—our kids—to make extra money." ◆

Studies That Connect Nutrition and Behavior

In the *Journal of Nutrition & Food Sciences*, Rausch (2013) article, "Nutrition and Academic Performance in School-Age Children," cites that nutritional deficiencies cause recognizable symptoms which disappear once the deficiency is alleviated. The research also showed that eating junk food decreases academic performance by limiting the amount of information to the brain.

The USDA Fruit and Vegetable Pilot Program found that teachers witnessed an increase in students' attention during class as a result of consuming an increased amount of fruits and vegetables. Similarly, studies of the School Breakfast Program Pilot Project found associations between participation in the breakfast program and better student behavior.

Research illustrates the need to help children maintain a nutrient-rich diet. Whether at home or at school, there is a responsibility to provide each child an equal chance to succeed academically, beginning with good nutrition.

In Conclusion

The story of Appleton Central Alternative High School proves that healthy food has a tremendous positive impact on mental health, emotional health, and academic performance.

CHAPTER 10
FOOD ALLERGIES AND
FOOD SENSITIVITIES

One person's poison, another person's medicine.

We have heard it said that one person's food is another person's poison, and that certainly applies to food allergies and food sensitivities!

Food Allergies and food sensitivities are a growing public health concern in the United States and are involved in many modern human illnesses. Food allergies can rev up the immune system and contribute to chronic inflammation. Although food sensitivities are more subtle than food allergies, they can also lead to many health problems.

More than 100 laws or regulations have been enacted by states in the last decade to address the needs of people with food allergies, according to the Food Allergy and Anaphylaxis Network, a nonprofit group. Awareness of food sensitivities has dramatically increased over the last decade. Even restaurants are posting information about food allergies in their kitchens and restaurant patrons now ask how foods are prepared and what ingredients are in their meals. Many restaurants even have special "gluten free" menus.

Discovering food sensitivities was an important part of our own healing journeys.

My Experience with Food Sensitivities—Sheri M.

The way I discovered my food sensitivities was on Monday mornings I'd often wake up with a headache and achy joints, my body feeling heavy and tired. I also felt like I had "brain fog," an inability to think clearly. I thought I just had "Monday morning blues" and for many years accepted this feeling as a normal part of my life. On the weekends I often attended potlucks, went out to restaurants, to friend's homes for dinner, or ate food that was catered. I ate whatever was being served without thinking much about it.

During the week when I had more control over my diet, I ate wholesome foods, but sometimes I had brain fog on weekdays, too. I didn't know why. After years of dealing with these symptoms, I began to make a connection between what I was eating and how I felt the next day. That's how I learned why Monday mornings were particularly difficult for me. Initially, it was hard to determine which foods were the culprit, but I got insight from going to a naturopathic doctor who used, among other techniques, muscle testing to determine which foods I was sensitive to. I also went to a practitioner who used NAET (Nambudripad's Allergy Elimination Technique) which employs Chinese meridian theory and uses homeopathic samples to test food allergies and sensitivities. This method was effective in reducing my symptoms of food sensitivities.

Once it was suspected that my reactions were from food sensitivities, I was able to notice which foods caused the problem. I started by eliminating gluten first, and soon had a reduction in my brain fog. This was a great revelation. What a relief to be able to think more clearly!

Then I began cutting down on sugar and cow dairy, and to my delight, I felt even better. An unexpected added bonus of cutting back on dairy was that my fall allergies of getting a runny nose and nasal congestion disappeared!

Next I eliminated MSG, additives, preservatives, and food coloring which I found had added to body aches and headaches. As I felt better and better, it became easier to avoid eating these foods because I wanted to feel good.

The next challenge was to still be able to attend potlucks and catered dinners, or go to restaurants and friend's homes for dinner without feeling bad the next day.

Following are tips on how I eat consciously and manage my food sensitivities when away from home:

1. **Potlucks.** I eat something at home before going that has some protein so I don't arrive too hungry. In addition, I bring a healthy dish that I know won't cause a food reaction.

The types of foods I gravitate toward at potlucks are usually a veggie platter, fruit salad or a green salad, and maybe some deli meats. I avoid dips or sauces because they often contain additives like preservatives and MSG. I may eat some plain corn chips and cheese. Although I have eliminated a lot of dairy, I find that I can now eat cow dairy occasionally and goat cheese without a problem.

If dessert is served, I find out if it's home-made or from a box. I stay away from grocery store cakes as they often contain a long list of ingredients including artificial flavorings, colorings, and additives that can ruin how I feel the next day. If the dessert is less processed, I will enjoy a small serving.

2. **Catered Meals.** I find out, if possible, who is catering the event and call to ask about the menu. Sometimes I'm able to speak with the chef for more details. Sometimes the caterer will even set aside a particular dish for me.

3. **Restaurants.** In recent years, restaurants have become more accommodating to people with food sensitivities and food allergies. By looking at the menu online or calling ahead, I can get an idea of options I will have upon arrival. Many restaurants are now including gluten-free and dairy-free items on their menus and more and more restaurants are eliminating the use of MSG.

When ordering a salad, I ask if the dressing is made at the restaurant or comes from a bottle. If they make their own, I find I can usually eat it without a problem. If it's bottled, I'll just ask for oil and vinegar on the side. (Bottled dressings often have preservatives and other additives).

4. **Dinner at a Friend's Home.** If I'm invited to dinner at a friend's home, I call the hostess ahead of time and let them know about my food sensitivities. This may seem like an extreme measure, but this way I can avoid any uncomfortable feelings on the part of the hostess or

myself if I arrive at their home and find I can't eat what they're serving. Friends hosting a party prefer to have something on hand that I can eat rather than me showing up and saying I can't eat what's being served.

5. **Carrying Snacks.** I always carry snacks such as gluten-free crackers, nuts, or a meal bar in my purse. This ensures I have a quick, healthy snack available at all times.

Discovering my food sensitivities and eliminating these foods from my diet has helped me become a more conscious eater and to feel more in control of my life and my health.

My motivation has been and will continue to be the desire to feel good, think more clearly, and have more energy. ◆

Discovering Food Sensitivities Was Key to Healing —Angie L.

For me, eliminating gluten, sugar (all forms except fruit, xylitol, and stevia), tomatoes, and coffee ultimately is what helped me manage and eventually reverse arthritis. These are the foods I used to eat all the time so giving them up wasn't easy. But when I looked at the alternative: taking drugs to manage inflammation or eliminating trigger foods to ease pain naturally, the choice to eliminate them was easier.

The first thing I eliminated was gluten, which was challenging because it seemed like it was in everything. The first thing I remember giving up was pizza. So whenever I went to an Italian restaurant or pizza place, I ordered an antipasto salad and skipped the bread. I used to love to eat crackers, cereal, and bread. During that time, there were not a lot of gluten-free options like there are today so I focused on oatmeal or eggs for breakfast, salads with chicken for lunch, and some sort of meat or fish and vegetables for dinner. I also supplemented my diet with a smoothie consisting of protein powder, rice milk, and banana or berries. This drink tasted delicious and helped me feel less deprived. It also boosted my energy because it was packed with vitamins and minerals.

Tomatoes were not as difficult to avoid and later I discovered that red peppers agreed with me so I learned how to substitute red peppers instead of tomatoes in omelets, stir fry, sauces and salads.

I first substituted coffee with a soy-based coffee then later learned to love a variety of teas. As I mention in the sugar chapter, I weaned myself off sugar by initially using artificial sugar and as I learned about the downside of artificial sweeteners I eventually discovered Stevia and have never looked back.

If I indulged in any of the foods I was sensitive to, I definitely noticed pain and inflammation in my fingers or toes.

By paying attention to how my body reacted to foods, it became apparent to me that giving up certain foods helped eliminate inflammation. As a result, I was able to go off my arthritis medication. Still to this day, this is how I manage arthritis. The reward of being pain-free is well worth my efforts!

Today I'm grateful for the variety of gluten-free options in breads, pasta, crackers, cereals, and even cookies. Using Stevia as a sweetener in making my own chocolate, muffins, and smoothies satisfies my sweet tooth. Now and then I still indulge in a "sugar-free" frozen yogurt as a special treat. Healthy grocery stores like Whole Foods carry chocolate bars sweetened with Stevia and frozen coconut chocolate bars sweetened with Erythritol.

It's not about giving up what you love but finding alternatives that work better for you. ♦

Here's a list of the most common foods that cause food sensitivities and/or food allergies:

gluten	sugar
dairy	soy
shellfish	citrus
tomatoes	corn
eggs	nuts
additives	MSG
food coloring	preservatives

Food Allergies and Food Sensitivities

There are two types of adverse reactions to food.

1. **The first type is a food allergy.** An allergy is severe and has immediate onset of symptoms such as anaphylactic shock, hives, swelling of skin, and asthma.

2. **The second type is a food sensitivity.** The distinction between food allergy and food sensitivity is that with a food sensitivity there may a delayed reaction. It is less severe than an allergy. Symptoms may appear within minutes, hours, or even the next day.

What is happening? An allergic reaction or sensitivity to food shifts the normal biochemistry to a status resembling a military red alert. The immune system is responding by mobilizing the body to reject the designated food. This can then boost levels of other substances, such as adrenaline and the stress hormone cortisol. Cells produce defense toxins to neutralize the invader. These toxins cause the side effects you experience. All of these stressful changes take a toll on the body and help deplete nutrients, so it is wise to reduce the symptoms of food allergies and sensitivities to relieve immediate discomfort and to lessen long-term wear and tear on your immune system. Symptoms of food allergies range from minor discomfort to life threatening anaphylactic shock such as a person's throat swelling when eating peanuts. The more often a food is eaten the more likely a person is to develop an allergy to it. Many people suffer from what is termed as an "Addictive/Allergic Response." This means that a person can actually be (and often is) allergic (or sensitive) to the foods they crave and they must eat these foods in order to not experience withdrawal symptoms such as headaches, leg cramps, fatigue, and lightheadedness.

Food allergy reactions are severe, immediate (two minutes to two hours) and can include:

- asthma
- difficulty breathing and/or anaphylaxis (throat swelling)
- drop in blood pressure or fainting
- hives
- vomiting

Food sensitivity (intolerance) reactions include a wide array of symptoms:

- tiredness/chronic fatigue
- coughing, irritated throat
- irritability
- joint and body aches
- headaches
- stiff neck
- poor concentration
- diarrhea/constipation
- asthma
- rhinitis (stuffed up nose)
- indigestion
- gas / bloating
- depression
- hyperactivity
- insomnia
- rashes/eczema
- feeling spacey or drugged
- poor balance
- inflammation (joints, skin)
- itching
- sleep disturbance
- agitation
- impatience
- mental confusion

Tyler's Corn and Chocolate Sensitivities—Laurie D.

When Tyler was two years old, he was dressed up for Halloween and helping pass out candy at our home. We had previously been told by our chiropractor that Tyler had a food allergy to corn that was creating a hyperactivity in him, as well as a predisposition to diabetes. So we had a homeopathic remedy administered to Tyler and eliminated all corn and corn derivatives, including corn syrup, from his diet. The calmness in him was noticeable and appreciated by me, his mom.

This particular evening, we made sure he did not eat any candy with corn in the ingredients but later that night, Tyler started coughing, violently. At about 5:00 a.m., I rushed him to the emergency room as he was still coughing and turning blue in the face. The doctors in the ER said he had whooping cough. I explained to them that Tyler had been vaccinated for whooping cough. They offered no remedy. So I took Tyler to our chiropractor at approximately 9:00 a.m.

Our chiropractor used applied kinesiology (muscle testing) and vials of food and in that methodical process, determined that Tyler was having an allergic reaction to chocolate. Halloween was the first time he had eaten chocolate in his young life. After a homeopathic remedy was given orally, the coughing stopped.

As the days ensued, to be safe, we eliminated chocolate from his diet, and the coughing did not return. Tyler is now eighteen years old and enjoys both corn and chocolate without any concerns or complaints or symptoms.

I was taught a valuable lesson that there are often many ways to heal that medically trained doctors may not be aware of and it is worth our time and effort and money to get to the root of an issue and remove the root cause so the symptom no longer presents itself. ◆

In Conclusion

We need to be mindful of how foods affect us. If we continually consume a food we are sensitive to, it can put unnecessary stress on the immune system that will weaken it over time, possibly leading to chronic or degenerative disease.

CHAPTER 11
GLUTEN SENSITIVITIES

I am eating gluten free because that little protein hurts my stomach, my joints, my muscles, and yes, even my brain.

Celiac Disease and Non-Celiac Gluten Sensitivity: More Common Than You Think

In recent years, people have become increasingly sensitive or allergic to gluten, the protein found in wheat, rye, barley, durum, semolina, spelt, Kamut®, farina, bulgur, couscous and "contaminated" oats (look for gluten-free oats if sensitive or allergic to gluten). The National Foundation for Celiac Awareness estimates that 18 million Americans have non-celiac gluten sensitivity. In *Going Against the Grain*, nutritionist Melissa Diane Smith writes that as many as half of Americans have some degree of gluten intolerance.

Approximately 3 million Americans have celiac disease. The gut damage from gluten can predispose people to numerous other food allergies. A damaged gut can allow undigested food proteins to enter the bloodstream, where they trigger an immune response.

There are a few reasons why gluten has become a health issue for so many people:

1. Hybridization has altered ancient wheat into a modern wheat. Modern wheat has been bred to contain more gluten, making it more difficult for many people to digest.

2. Overconsumption of gluten can create a sensitivity or allergy.

3. Food manufacturers flavor foods with added sugar, high fructose corn syrup, salt, and many other unnecessary and unhealthy additives.

4. Gluten-containing grains contain gliadin molecules that can cause an immune response and damage surrounding tissue.

A true gluten allergy is a serious condition known as celiac disease. Celiac disease is far less common than non-celiac gluten sensitivity. If you have been suffering symptoms that seem related to gluten but tested negative for celiac disease, it may be possible that you have non-celiac gluten sensitivity.

Celiac Disease

Celiac disease is an autoimmune condition to which the body can't process gluten. For people with celiac disease or undiagnosed non-celiac gluten sensitivity, ingesting even tiny amounts of gluten can set off an autoimmune reaction that flattens the finger-like villi lining the small intestine. Even ketchup and soy sauce may contain gluten or wheat. Reading labels is a must for those with celiac disease or celiac intolerance. People that are sensitive to gluten can also be sensitive to casein. Casein makes up about 80% of the proteins present in cow's milk.

Non-celiac gluten sensitivity is diagnosed by process of exclusion. If symptoms improve on a gluten-free diet, then you likely have non-celiac gluten sensitivity (or celiac disease). There are other alternative methods for testing for food sensitivities which are detailed later in this chapter.

Symptoms of Celiac Disease or Non-Celiac Gluten Sensitivity

abdominal pain	gas / bloating
diarrhea	constipation
irritable bowel syndrome	coughing
brain fog	migraine headaches
early osteoporosis	anemia
bone and joint pain	chronic fatigue
dental problems	peripheral neuropathy
seizures	elevated liver enzymes
easy bruising of skin	behavioral problems
unexplained infertility	diabetes
depression	neurological problems
liver problems	rapid heartbeat
fatigue	throat irritation

Below Peter shares an inspiring story about his gluten sensitivity.

My Gluten Sensitivity Story—Peter F.

In the 1970s, I became motivated to improve the quality of my diet because of several influences.

First, the fabulous Jack LaLanne, famous fitness guru, came to our high school and gave a lecture about the wonders of good nutrition and exercise. Second, a friend of mine on the track team turned me onto Bob Hoffman vitamins and supplements. Then and there, I became hooked on health foods and healthy living. My journey to health had begun.

I investigated and experimented with many diets and exercise programs and became a vegetarian. I fell back into the Standard American Diet for a two-to-three-year period in the 1980s and started developing problems with my intestines.

Eventually, with a desire to improve my health, I got on a vegan diet in the last years of the 1980s. I was very enthusiastic about my diet but things started to go downhill for me. I became more and more constipated, even though I was eating massive amounts of fiber in the form of fruits, vegetables, whole grains, whole grain breads and crackers, beans, legumes, nuts, and seeds. I also had little energy and began to have joint problems which limited the amount of running I could do. This loss alone was emotionally devastating. How could this be happening?

It would take the entire next decade and a bit more to find out.

In the 1990s, my wife and I enthusiastically embarked on a series of herbal cleansing programs. With the positive results we were getting, I was joyfully optimistic and felt we had discovered the missing piece of the health puzzle. After four years of herbal cleansing programs, I decided to take a break. So, I followed a new diet I discovered (Fit for Life) and began to exercise almost every day with running and walking. After one more cleansing process, things starting to go seriously downhill. In 1995, I noticed a bulge growing in my right groin. This steadily got worse and my energy started going downhill, too. What was going on? I was doing all the "right things"—good diet and exercise.

During the last half of the 1990s, I tried many diets and programs plus even more herbal cleansing, but to no avail. My intestines got worse, with lots of gas, pain, and continued constipation. Everything I knew from the past that I trusted seemed to not be working. I got really desperate, willing to try anything.

With a lot of prayer, help came in several unexpected directions. First, I discovered feng shui, Chinese life force energy balancing. I gradually cleaned up the external mess that I had created because of my poor health and low energy. This led me, through a friend, to the Specific Carbohydrate Diet (SCD). It seemed very restricted and different. But I was very motivated to stick to the program and stop the almost constant intestinal pain, gas, constipation and low energy.

The SCD helped me tremendously over the next few years. This diet eliminates all grains, most starches, refined sugars, and many dairy products containing lactose (milk sugar).

It took over a year to start feeling better but my symptoms gradually went away.

I later discovered that it was the absence of gluten, a protein found in wheat, rye, barley, and spelt that was what made the SCD work for me.

In 2002, I also found that by combining the SCD with the Blood Type Diet my health improved even more. Now that I was gluten-free, I could do the exercise that I loved to do such as running, hiking, rock climbing, backpacking, and cycling with no pain.

By getting off gluten, and combining healing modalities plus prayer, I was able to heal myself.

Today, at the age of sixty, I have a full life, and a good career as a massage therapist, reflexologist, and nutrition/health consultant. I run marathons and also have a career as a musician and teacher.

I'm happy to share my story because I think a lot of people can benefit from being gluten-free. ♦

Below is Don's story that illustrates how gluten can cause varied symptoms written by Don Ellison, author of *The Acts of Creation: A Workbook for Adults Who Work or Live with Children and Young Adults, to Teach Them Intuitive, Psychic and Spiritual Science Skills.*

Why I Got Off Gluten—Don E.

In my mid-fifties, I was having violent coughing spells that prompted me to go to the doctor. I was diagnosed with an allergy to pollen or chemicals in the air. I started using Qbar and Albuterol to counteract the coughing. It worked pretty well for a while, but I found myself using it more frequently. I had heard from other friends that this was not a good thing for my health in the long run.

One day, talking with a friend, I learned that I could alleviate allergic symptoms by getting off of dairy; I did. It worked for a couple of years and eventually, the cough came back. Well, this time I decided to take matters in my own hands and use my pendulum (which I have used for about twenty-five years) to determine the reason for my continued coughing spells.

My coughing got pretty violent at times and I found I couldn't breathe until I took a puff of my inhaler. As I worked with my pendulum, I determined I was allergic to wheat (gluten).

I stopped consuming wheat and my coughing lessoned until it stopped altogether. I rarely have to take a puff of my inhaler these days. I also found by cutting back on sweets, I could alleviate any other allergic problems altogether. ◆

In Conclusion

Ironically, by repeatedly eating the same foods you can create sensitivities to them. There may be certain foods you crave often, such as pasta, bread and cereal, for example. Many people are sensitive and/or allergic to gluten without realizing it. We recommend abstaining for one week from gluten and notice how you feel. If you feel noticeably better, you may have a gluten sensitivity.

CHAPTER 12
DAIRY AND OTHER SENSITIVITIES

Just because we have been doing it for centuries,
does not mean it is rational or good for us; it just means it
was an available food source at some point, and has
since become an acceptable part of the human diet.

Dairy & Lactose Intolerance

It is estimated that 30 to 50 million Americans suffer from some form of dairy intolerance. Pasteurized cow's milk is the number one allergic food in the United States. It has been associated with a number of symptoms and illnesses including:

- diarrhea, cramps, bloating, and gas
- nasal congestion
- osteoporosis
- arthritis
- heart disease
- recurrent ear infections and colic in infants and children
- type 1 diabetes
- rheumatoid arthritis
- infertility
- autism

Many people have a dairy intolerance due to lactose (milk sugar) without even realizing it. Others have a dairy allergy to milk protein.

Lactose occurs naturally in the milk of animals. Many people are sensitive to milk products because they lack the enzyme called lactase. This enzyme, found in the gastrointestinal tract, is critical in the digestion of lactose. If the lactase enzyme is missing or depleted, the gastrointestinal tract cannot adequately break down the milk sugar, leading to a wide variety of symptoms. When this occurs, these individuals are described as being lactose intolerant. Symptoms from lactose intolerance can vary greatly from one individual to the next as well as vary within the individual. Some people find that taking lactase enzymes helps digest the lactose.

Symptoms of Lactose Intolerance

These symptoms include but are not limited to:

- stomach cramps
- intestinal bloating or "pot belly"
- flatulence
- diarrhea
- headaches
- nausea

Dairy Allergy

As with the symptoms of lactose intolerance, the reaction to milk proteins can also vary greatly from one individual to the next. When the immune system recognizes the milk proteins whey and casein as being harmful, this creates the dairy allergy. This response can intensify over time, particularly if dairy is continually consumed.

Symptoms of Dairy Allergy

Dairy allergy symptoms tend to increase in severity from that of lactose intolerance. These symptoms include but are not limited to:

- stomach cramps
- intestinal bloating or "pot belly"
- flatulence
- diarrhea
- constipation
- headaches
- nausea
- asthma
- nasal congestion or mucous buildup
- skin rash
- hives
- fatigue
- eczema

- bleeding from the bowel
- rectal fissures
- rectal itching
- anaphylactic shock

My Dairy Sensitivity Story—Sheri M.

I discovered my dairy sensitivities in a very odd way. I was having nasal congestion every Fall. I knew I didn't have a cold and I couldn't figure out why I was congested. This went on for several seasons.

Then one Fall, I decided to try getting off dairy foods to see if my achy joints got better. Low and behold, not only did my joint pain improve, my nasal congestion completely disappeared! Now I avoid dairy and continue to enjoy the benefits. ♦

Goat Dairy

The good news is that many people who cannot tolerate cow dairy can often times tolerate goat products. Goat products such as milk, cheese, yogurt, and kefir are easier to digest than dairy from cows. Goat milk is more digestible because the fat molecules are one-fifth the size of those from cow milk—making it easily tolerated by those with compromised digestive systems.

A few other facts about goat milk:

- Seventy-two percent of the milk used throughout the world is from goats. It is one-third richer than cow milk, is more nourishing, and easier to digest.
- Goat milk is closer to human milk and is therefore easily accepted especially by those young or frail.
- Goat milk has an alkaline reaction the same as mother's milk. Cow milk has an acid reaction.
- Goat milk does not form mucous (phlegm) and is therefore better tolerated by asthmatics and those with allergies.
- Goat milk has the ability to soothe the intestinal tract and assist with constipation.

Kefir

Now a few words about kefir. Kefir can be made from cows or goats. It is a cultured, creamy product with various health attributes. For all the health benefits listed above regarding goat dairy, we recommend goat over cow kefir, especially for those who are sensitive to cow dairy.

Kefir's creamy and refreshing flavor is similar to a yogurt drink, and it contains beneficial yeast, bacteria, and lactase, an enzyme which consumes most of the lactose left after the culturing process. It is similar to the beneficial yeast and bacteria provided by lactase. The naturally occurring bacteria and yeast in kefir combine symbiotically to give superior health benefits. It is loaded with valuable vitamins and minerals and contains easily digestible complete proteins.

There are now many wonderful dairy alternatives such as almond milk, rice milk, or coconut milk available at most grocery stores.

Food Additives

Some people may be more sensitive to chemicals added to food than the food itself. This is where it can get tricky to determine the culprit of your symptom(s). If you have a reaction after eating, note whether the food you consumed listed any of these additives as ingredients. They may be the hidden cause for your food reaction. Here are examples of such food additives:

- Monosodium glutamate (MSG)
- Preservatives
- Nitrites or nitrates
- Food coloring
- Food additives
- Sulfur dioxide or sulfites

Keep in mind processed foods contain many of these types of chemicals.

Excitotoxins: A Downright Dangerous Additive

What do monosodium glutamate (MSG), hydrolyzed vegetable protein, and aspartame (NutraSweet, the substance in Diet Coke and diet Red Bull) have in common? They are common taste-enhancing additives found in a variety of foods and beverages, and they all contain excitotoxins. In his book, *Excitotoxins: The Taste That Kills*, Dr. Russell L. Blaylock provides an extensive review of the literature supporting his claim that these excitatory amino acids can promote the death of neurons in the brain and spinal cord. Dr. Blaylock defines excitotoxins as a group of amino acids that can cause sensitive neurons to die. The most common ones are glutamate, aspartame, and cysteine.

Although excitotoxins are widely distributed in our food supply, Dr. Blaylock points out that we may not be able to depend upon the Food and Drug Administration (FDA) to protect us from these toxic amino acids. It's up to us to read labels and limit consumption of these additives.

Losing Weight and Food Sensitivities

Discovering your food sensitivities and allergies can also help you lose weight because when you eat a food you're sensitive to, it causes a series of negative biochemical reactions in your system and digestive tract that can hinder your weight loss efforts. It also decreases your serotonin levels and can make you feel slightly depressed, causing you to turn to sugars and simple carbohydrates for relief. Medical intuitive Caroline Sutherland, in her book, *How to Crack the Weight Loss Code*, believes strongly that food sensitivities are responsible for the majority of people's inability to lose weight and crack their own weight loss code.

Many people are sensitive to wheat, gluten, dairy, and sugar and could reduce health issues by eliminating these foods.

Testing for Food Allergies or Sensitivities

We recommend that you begin to pay attention to how you feel immediately after eating, hours later, or even the next day. You may notice physical symptoms such as a runny nose, the need to clear your throat often, brain fog, joint aches, or headaches. Making the connection between a symptom and a food can save you a lifetime of frustration, medication, and doctor visits. There are no standard tests used to confirm or rule out a food allergy. Your doctor may do some testing or make a referral to an allergy specialist.

1. **Skin test.** A skin prick test can determine your reaction to a particular food. Keep in mind, a positive reaction to this test alone isn't enough to confirm a food allergy.

2. **Blood tests.** Keep in mind that these testing methods are not always accurate.

- An IgE response (globulin responsible for allergic reactions) indicates an immediate reaction as with a food allergy.
- An IgG response indicates a delayed response as with a food sensitivity.
- RAST is used to determine the amount of IgE antibodies to the specific foods suspected of causing allergic reactions.
- IgG Elisa tests the antibody reaction to determine delayed food reactions (those occurring more than twenty-four hours after eating foods that trigger a reaction).

3. **Oral food challenge.** During this test, done in the doctor's office, you'll be given small, but increasing amounts of the suspect food. If you don't have a reaction during this test, you may be able to include this food in your diet again.

4. **Elimination diet.** You may be asked to eliminate suspect foods for a week or two, and then add the food items back into your diet one at a time. This process can help link symptoms to specific foods.

One of the best things you can do if you believe you are suffering from a food allergy is to do an elimination diet on your own:

- For two weeks, eliminate one food to give it a full trial.
- Try eliminating gluten first.
- If the symptoms disappear within a few days, it's safe to assume you have a sensitivity.
- If symptoms persist, try eliminating one at a time: dairy, corn, soy, eggs, peanuts, sugar, alcohol, preservatives, food coloring, artificial sweeteners, and/or caffeine.

Although an elimination diet can seem restrictive and difficult at first, you can still pack your grocery cart with plenty of nutritious, delicious food. You may be amazed at the results. In some cases you will eventually be able to slowly reintroduce offending foods back into your diet over time or have them just occasionally.

5. **Rotation Diet.** You can also try a rotation diet. Avoid eating the same food or foods from the same family (such as dairy) more often than once every four days. This allows the immune system time to recover.

6. **Nambudripad's Allergy Elimination Test (NAET).** Nambudripad's allergy elimination technique, also known as NAET, is a safe, effective, natural approach to detecting and eliminating all types of allergies. NAET combines techniques from kinesiology (muscle strength testing), chiropractic, and Oriental medicine, to clear allergic reaction through a "reprogramming" of the brain. If a muscle goes weak while you hold a certain food, this can indicate a food sensitivity. The actual technique used involves light acupressure applied along both sides of the spinal column in an area where the energy flow of a meridian intersects with the nerve roots.

In Conclusion

Many people are sensitive and/or allergic to wheat, gluten, dairy and sugar without realizing it. You can reduce health issues by finding alternatives to these foods.

Each person is different. Once you discover foods that you are allergic or sensitive to, it will be up to you to avoid them. Then notice how you feel, and slowly introduce them back into your diet. You may realize you feel better without certain foods altogether, as was the case with both of us.

CHAPTER 13
SUGAR AND ITS MANY DISGUISES

Sugar is the most dangerous drug of our time and
should come with smoking-style health warnings.
—Paul van der Velpen
Head of Amsterdam Health Services

If you do a Google search on "sugar harmful effects to body" you will literally get millions of results about the harmful effects of sugar.

As delicious as all those sweets are, experts agree that refined sugar acts more like a pharmaceutical drug in the body than a nurturing food.

Sugar has many names on labels. A few examples are high fructose corn syrup (HFCS), dextrose, glucose, fructose, maltose, evaporated cane juice, and Sucanat. According to brain specialist Dr. Daniel Amen, "They are all bad for your brain and health."

The good news is that once you've broken your sugar addiction, you will feel dramatically better and your body should be able to handle sugar in moderation.

Sugar: Then and Now

At the beginning of this century, two-thirds of the carbohydrates eaten by Americans came from complex sources such as potatoes, vegetables, and grains. The World Health Organization recommends we consume only 10% from simple sources (sugars). The reality is about 60% of all carbohydrates we consume come from simple sugars and simple carbohydrates. The human body was never designed to deal with this many simple sugars.

The far-reaching problems sugar can cause are well-documented in medical journals throughout the world and new disease connections are made each year. Take for example heart disease, cancer, and diabetes, the three leading disease killers in the U.S. today. Although the media has presented bad fats (such as hydrogenated or partially hydrogenated oil) as the villain in the development of these diseases, sugar appears to be the other culprit.

We expect sugar to be in foods like cakes, cookies, candy, sodas, donuts, jellies, and desserts, but now it shows up in unexpected foods such as bread, salad dressings, pickles, mayonnaise, ketchup, tomato sauce, baby food, frozen fruit, cereal, canned vegetables, packaged meat, and the list goes on. No wonder we've become so addicted to sugar! Manufacturers of processed food have contributed to our loss of appetite for natural, whole foods and our ability to appreciate the sweetness of a carrot, a sweet potato, or green peas by adding various sugars and salt to most packaged foods.

To understand what sugar really is, you first have to understand some basics about carbohydrates. Carbohydrates are one of the three energy producing nutrients our bodies need. The other two are protein and fat.

The two types of carbohydrates are:

1. **Simple carbohydrates.** When simple carbs are eaten, they are broken down almost immediately, and a flood of sugar is released directly into the bloodstream. When digesting simple carbs, insulin levels spike faster, and the carb is used more quickly. Grains such as white rice and white pasta are processed as a simple carb which breaks down in the body like sugar. This explains why your energy is up and then crashes after eating sugar and refined carbs. This spike in energy is what makes simple carbs so addicting.

If your cells are filled with fat and sugar, they cannot respond appropriately to insulin. This forces the pancreas to make many times the normal amount of insulin in an effort to stimulate your cells to respond. High insulin causes some of your sugar to be stored as fat. The increased body fat causes insulin resistance and prevents glucose from entering your cells. This sustained high insulin levels leads to insulin resistance contributing to diabetes, obesity, and heart disease.

2. **Complex Carbohydrates.** These are more complex in structure and take longer to digest. Because the sugars are released more slowly and gradually into the bloodstream, they supply steadier, longer-lasting energy for the body. These wholesome carbs contain beneficial vitamins, minerals, fiber, and antioxidants and are metabolized more slowly than simple carbs. Complex carbs are vegetables, legumes (beans), and whole grains such as brown or wild rice, quinoa, sprouted breads, oatmeal, and whole grain cereals.

In addition to sugar, another sweetener of great concern is high fructose corn syrup (HFCS). Dr. Robert Lustig, Neuroendocrinologist and Professor with the Department of Epidemiology and Metabolism at UCSF, has dedicated his lectures to focus on the health threat of sugar, namely in the form of HFCS. He says, "If you want to lose weight, [and] avoid diabetes and heart disease, you want to avoid sugar, especially in the form of HFCS. Sucrose (sugar) and fructose (specifically HFCS) are equally bad, poisonous, dangerous." HFCS also raises your triglycerides and LDL (bad cholesterol) and is more readily metabolized to fat in the liver than glucose. This leads to insulin resistance. Another concern is that HFCS is almost always made from genetically modified corn, which has its own side effects.

The Corn Refiners Association (CRA) has resorted to creating a new label for HFCS by calling it "fructose syrup" or just "fructose" because numerous studies have linked HFCS to obesity, type 2 diabetes and autism. Psychology professor Bart Hoebel of Princeton University reports, "When rats are drinking HFCS at levels well below those in soda pop, they're becoming obese; every single one, across the board. Even when rats are fed a high-fat diet, you don't see this; they don't all gain extra weight."

It may not always be easy, but to give you some ideas, we share our stories below to tell what worked for us to kick the sugar habit. Some of these ideas may be helpful or you may find other ways that work better for you.

How I Licked My Sugar Habit—Angie L.

I have always had a sweet tooth. My earliest memory of "sweet" is eating bread, milk, and syrup for breakfast with my three siblings at the kitchen table at our red house in Houston, Texas. We weren't poor, but there were many mouths to feed and we were all big eaters. We probably went through an entire loaf of bread at the first meal of the day! I was about three years old.

When my family moved to Southern California, I was ten years old and loved to ride my skateboard with friends to the Redondo Beach pier. We would pick out handfuls of candies from the large barrels at the candy story. My other pleasure was eating large marshmallows, one right after another, after school.

In middle school I lived in South Dakota. My best friend, Shelley, and I loved sports. We also loved sweets. Immediately after school we would stop at The Shack snack shop near the school to load up on candy bars, sodas, Skittles, Snickers, you name it. We were both very active so weight wasn't an issue. But by the time I was sixteen, my entire mouth had been filled with dental fillings—proof that sugar leads to tooth decay.

In high school I loved to stop by The Bread Box bakery on Main Street, just a block away from my home on my way to school. We lived so close you could smell the aroma of cinnamon and bread baking. I would buy a cinnamon roll, a maple bar, or glazed donut. Sugar was always on my mind and my mom made sure there was plenty in the house. My mother and my Uncle Lyle loved to bake brownies, cookies, bars, pies, and cakes. We always had a couple tins of baked goods on the kitchen counter free for the taking. Eating goodies like this occasionally is okay but not on a daily basis. It never, ever occurred to me that sugar may not be good for me.

When I developed arthritis, I began noticing that when I did eat sugar, I would feel pain in my joints within a few minutes and my skin would also flare in the form of psoriasis. I started to make the connection between sugar and inflammation. I think all those years of sugar contributed to weakening my immune system and these reactions were my body's way of saying "No thank you, I've had enough."

So I slowly weaned myself off sugar by doing more artificial sugar in the form of Diet Coke and began to sweeten everything with artificial sweeteners. Then I began to learn about artificial sweeteners and all the problems they can cause. Eventually I decided to go off all artificial sweeteners and refined sugar because I did not want to put chemicals in my body.

I don't feel deprived in my life now because I have discovered other healthier alternatives to sugar, namely Stevia, which you will learn more about in this chapter. I make my own muffins, coconut bars, and even chocolates with Stevia. I've found that I can be just as satisfied with these baked goods without the ill side effects from processed and artificial sugar.

Getting off refined sugar (and artificial sugar) was a process that took me several years because the taste of sweet is very addicting. The motivating factor for me was that these foods caused physical pain in my joints, namely in my fingers and toes. When I was masking the arthritis with pain meds, I couldn't determine which foods were increasing inflammation. But once I went off them, it became very obvious that sugar (and gluten) created pain and inflammation in my body. This made me a more mindful eater.

For the five years between giving up artificial sugar and discovering Stevia, I abstained from all forms of desserts and sweets with the exception of fruit.

Another effect that sugar had on me was hyperglycemia. When I stopped eating so many carbs and sugar and added more protein to my diet, I no longer experienced that weak, shaky feeling. Eliminating refined sugars helped to balance my blood sugar, energy level, weight, mood, hormones, and frankly, all aspects of my life.

Being pain-free and having my body and mind in balance makes being sugar-free worth it. With healthy sweeteners like Stevia, Erythritol and Xylitol, I no longer feel deprived like I once did.

Recently, a friend brought potato salad for a barbeque I was hosting. I did not inquire about ingredients; I simply enjoyed a good-sized portion of potato salad. The next day I had pain in my finger joints. So I looked at the ingredients from the left-over (store-bought) potato salad since it was still in its original container in my refrigerator. Sugar was listed five times...in potato salad! Even I was surprised. So we get sugar even when we're not craving it or expecting it. The pain in my fingers subsided within a couple days, but these are my occasional reminders for me to stay away from sugar. Ultimately, it's about finding balance for each of us, staying healthy and as pain-free as possible. ♦

My Sugar Story—Sheri M.

My first relationship with sugar began when I was a little girl at the age of four in Cleveland, Ohio. My family would often take Sunday drives to Chagrin Falls. We drove over a little bridge and then went to an old-fashioned ice cream parlor with red leather stools. The smell of ice cream filled the air. My favorite was vanilla and I relished licking my vanilla ice cream cone as we walked around and looked at the waterfalls. Vanilla ice cream has remained, to this day, my favorite sweet treat.

Growing up, we had dessert for special occasions like birthdays, but our usual sweet after dinner was fruit. My family would sit and watch TV and my mom brought in a big bowl of whatever fruit was in season. I particularly loved green grapes, and I would stuff them in my mouth like a little squirrel. I can still taste the sweet juice as it burst into my mouth.

As a teenager, I would occasionally buy a twenty-five-cent snail roll on our "nutrition break." This consisted of cinnamon and sugar between a circle of folds of flour. I always felt a little guilty buying these as I knew my mom didn't want us to eat too many sweets. She had learned from some relatives and from reading books on healthy eating that limiting desserts and junk food was important for the health of her family.

When I got married and had two sons of my own, I made special cakes for them on their birthdays. One example was a fire engine cake, made out of bricks of strawberry ice cream with red licorice and gumdrops for decoration. On their birthday, they could choose whatever cereal they wanted (Fruit Loops were a favorite) and whatever dessert they wanted in their school lunch. My kids knew dessert was only for a special occasion and I prided myself in raising them this way.

Although I didn't know details of the negative effects of sugar, I knew that a balanced diet low in sugar and high in vegetables and fruit was the best way to eat. The hard part was going to parties and friends' homes and especially at Halloween time. Put all those goodies in front of me and I have a hard time resisting! Tootsie rolls and chocolate bars were my first choice. Eating these sweets would start the sugar craving cycle making it difficult to resist. Eventually I would get back to eating healthy and the cravings would eventually subside. The key for me was not having tempting sweets in the house.

Skipping to the present day, I still love sweets and desserts but have come to learn the effects sugar has on me. I learned this through dealing with ulcerative colitis and Lyme disease as sugar exacerbates both of these conditions. I've learned to incorporate what I call the 90/10 rule and indulge in treats only on very special occasions. (This means 90% of the time I focus on eating highly nutritious foods which I truly do enjoy, and the other 10% I allow myself some treats at birthdays, parties, and other special occasions.) This really works for me.

In addition to knowing sugar was not good for me, the other motivation was noticing that I would initially feel good when eating it, but soon after, my energy level would drop and I then felt tired. I didn't like that feeling. I also learned that sugar caused spikes in my blood sugar and it put my body out of balance. Sometimes I had brain fog. Other times, I felt achy or irritable. I could always trace it back to sugar I had eaten recently, such as desserts at friend's homes or even a chai tea latte.

To begin the process of giving up sugar, I made sure I didn't have sweets in the house. If they were in front of me I was too easily tempted. It was not easy at first. I learned to substitute fruit even though fruit is high in sugar. Apples and berries were a good choice since the fiber helped the fruit sugar metabolize more slowly.

After being off sugar for about a week, the cravings were much less. Within a few weeks I didn't miss it that much. I did have to be careful in those initial stages to not overdo sugar at a special occasion. I would either stay away from it or have just a bite or two. Otherwise, because sugar is so addictive, the craving cycle would be reactivated.

Today, to satisfy sweet cravings, I often make a smoothie for breakfast or a snack using hempseed, rice milk or coconut milk, protein powder, sometimes kefir, a handful of berries, and a tablespoon of nut butter such as almond or sunflower butter, vanilla, and a couple drops of Stevia. I also use Stevia to sweeten my tea.

If I desire something sweet after a meal, I'll have a couple squares of dark chocolate or some coconut milk with a drop or two of Stevia and yum, I feel like my need for something sweet has been satisfied. ♦

Giving Up Sugar to Reverse Arthritis, Fatigue, and Eczema—Ron H.

I suffered from bouts of eczema, arthritis, and fatigue for ten years until I seriously started to change my diet.

My problems with eczema started at the age of eleven with a bad case on my ankles. After our regular doctor's creams didn't help, my thoughtful mother took me to a "health foods" doctor, who said to eliminate sugar, fats, and carbs, and recommended my mother serve more fresh fruits and vegetables, boil greens to drink the cleansing liquid, and eat lots of garlic.

In retrospect, that doctor's understanding of the nutritional connection to the body was way ahead of his time.

Even though my mother mindfully prepared good, healthy meals, which I enjoyed, my desire for sweets only increased.

So, in my middle and high school years when I was alone out on my bike, I snuck a lot of candy and sugary drinks, to fill that desire for sweets. I could tell you what every candy bar tasted like.

As the years progressed, I became more aware of the fatigue I felt after eating a small amount of orange juice or baked goods. My doctor said that, besides my high cholesterol, my blood sugar level was dangerously high.

He also said that the developing arthritis in my shoulder and arm was "natural aging" and suggested Tylenol.

I knew I had enough with all the pain and fatigue. I had to get real serious about controlling my highly imbalanced diet and food lifestyle. I wanted to be done having food hangovers and arthritis in my arms and shoulders.

I am fortunate to have the wisdom of the old "health-foods" doctor of my childhood, and the wonderful influences of my mother's healthy food practices to help motivate me.

I am also fortunate to know Sheri Miller, who is very knowledgeable about diet. Our discussions about health issues have significantly informed my understanding about a smart, healthy food lifestyle.

I had to dig deep and focus to stay on point.

I was able to gradually stop eating sugar, gluten, dairy, and red meat, because my efforts to control my food resulted in feeling much better, and my blood panel test read in the "normal range."

My current diet is basically: chicken, fish, turkey, beans, vegetables, fruit, and nuts, and I never feel cheated because I feel so much better! But that doesn't mean that I'm "perfect' in my diet because I'm not, and I don't try to be.

For me, I've found that if I "eat right" for a period of time, I can have some sort of a treat and not feel any or little food hangover the next day.

It is a matter of balance for me to feel well and have control over my health. ♦

Tips to Kick the Sugar Habit

1. **Begin gradually** and do a slow transition. First, eliminate the sugars you are not likely to miss, like sugar hidden in drinks or in convenience foods.

2. **Limit your consumption of refined sugar products** such as cookies, cakes, donuts, white bread, white rice, white pasta, and bagels.

3. **Include more complex carbohydrates** in your diet: brown rice, whole grain breads, oatmeal, millet, quinoa, fruits, and vegetables.

4. **Eat unprocessed whole foods** to cut down on your sugar intake: fish, poultry, meat, eggs, grains, nuts, and legumes. Fruits and vegetables are full of fiber and nutrients, which help balance blood sugar.

5. **Reduce amount of sugar** in recipes. As a sugar substitute use stevia, brown rice syrup, xylitol, or erythritol.

6. **Use a drop or two of Stevia or Xylitol** if you need to sweeten tea or cereal. These are natural sweeteners that won't spike your blood sugar.

7. **Read nutrition labels** closely. Buy products with the least amount of grams of sugar. Eventually the goal is to buy foods with less than five grams of sugar per serving. Remember, stevia, xylitol, or erythritol are basically zero grams of sugar.

8. **Write down what you eat**. This will raise awareness of your patterns of eating. For example, a breakfast of toast, jelly, and orange juice starts a cycle of sugar swings and sugar cravings.

9. **Eat protein and good fats at every meal**. This keeps your blood sugar balanced which helps with mood and energy levels.

10. **Practice moderation with caffeine**. Excess caffeine can result in blood sugar imbalance and lead to sugar cravings.

11. **Drink clean water.** Craving sweets can be a sign of dehydration. Drink a glass of water and notice if this helps with cravings.

12. **Use healthy alternatives to sugar.** Use sweeteners like Stevia, brown rice syrup, Xylitol, and Erythritol instead of sugar.

13. **Get your body moving.** Begin with walking or yoga. Exercise will help balance your blood sugar levels and reduce stress.

14. **Try using spices.** The natural sweetness of coriander, cinnamon, nutmeg, cloves, and cardamom can satisfy sweet cravings.

15. **Get good sleep.** Lack of sleep, going to bed late, or waking up early can cause sugar cravings.

16. **Talk to your physician if you're on medication**. If you cut down on sugar, your blood pressure or cholesterol meds may need to be reduced and even eliminated.

Food Tips: 20 Healthy Ways to Satisfy Your Sweet Cravings

1. Apple slices (or celery sticks) with sunflower or almond butter topped with a few raisins

2. Baked apple with 1/4 cup chopped nuts, sprinkled with raisins, and a pinch of cinnamon and nutmeg. Add 1/4 cup water to the pan and bake at 350° for 20 minutes.

3. Smoothie made with rice, almond, hemp, or coconut milk, goat kefir, or yogurt, protein powder, half a banana, spinach or kale, and a couple drops of Stevia for added sweetness

4. Goat yogurt or goat kefir topped with berries and nuts (sweeten with a couple drops of Stevia or Xylitol)

5. Unsweetened cereal with rice, almond, hemp, coconut, goat milk, or goat kefir and a handful of almonds or walnuts. Sweeten with Stevia or Xylitol.

6. Cut up banana and freeze; it tastes like banana ice cream

7. Muffins made with almond flour or coconut flour; use Stevia or Xylitol as sugar substitutes

8. Mixed nuts and seeds with raisins and goji berries or raw cacao nibs

9. Baked sweet potato with coconut oil

10. Ground flaxseed in almond milk with Stevia or Xylitol

11. Tahini butter (or any other nut or seed butter) with Stevia

12. Coconut milk with a couple drops of Stevia

13. Herbal teas with Stevia or Xylitol

14. Sparkling water with Stevia or Xylitol and lemon

15. Spry gum or mints sweetened with Xylitol at Whole Foods or a health food store

16. Mix raw cacao powder in warm almond or coconut milk with a couple drops of Stevia

17. Drink coconut water. It's naturally sweet and very hydrating.

18. Make your own chocolates with raw cacao, coconut oil, and Stevia.

19. Mixed fruit salad with nuts. Fruit gets metabolized as sugar but has healthy fiber and nutrients. Limit your fruit intake to one to two fruits a day.

20. Stock healthful, easy-to-grab foods free of sugar for sudden cravings. Examples: nuts, whole-grain crackers, and cheese.

Note: Xylitol is a sugar alcohol and some people react with gas or bloating. For these reasons, Stevia is our first choice for a healthy sugar alternative.

What Is Your Relationship to Sugar?

Do you struggle with eating too much sugar? Or are you someone who enjoys it in moderation? In a journal or notebook, take some time to write down your favorite type of sweet and your memories around it. This exercise may help you understand your emotional connection to sugar. Remember, each person is different and has varying tolerance levels for sugar.

Here's an abbreviated list of conditions that can be caused by consuming too much sugar:

- adrenal gland exhaustion
- alcoholism
- allergies
- anxiety

- arthritis
- asthma
- behavior problems
- binge eating
- bone loss
- candida
- cancer
- colitis
- constipation
- depression
- diabetes
- difficulty concentrating
- fatigue
- food cravings
- high blood pressure
- hyperactivity
- insomnia
- mood swings
- obesity
- tooth decay
- yeast infections

Sugar Facts

1. According to the American Medical Association, we now consume at least 140 pounds of sugar per person per year which translates to about twenty-two teaspoons of added sugar a day for adults and thirty-four teaspoons a day for teens.

2. Sugar is a known immune suppressant. It has been proven to destroy the germ-killing ability of white blood cells for up to five hours after ingestion.

3. Type 2 diabetes has increased dramatically with the increase of sugar consumption.

4. If cells become cancerous, they feed directly on sugar and sugar can accelerate tumor growth.

5. Sugar intake is linked to depression and mood swings.

6. Sugar increases insulin. Sustained high insulin levels can lead to insulin resistance contributing to diabetes, obesity, and heart disease.

7. Cells have a limited capacity for sugar. An excess will be stored as fat which leads to weight gain.

8. Overconsumption of sugar over time can cause your pancreas to "burn out" from having to secrete large amounts of insulin.

9. Sugar causes you to lose important minerals. As little as two tablespoons of sugar disturbs delicate mineral ratios.

10. Reducing refined carbs and eliminating refined sugars from your diet protects your body from storing fat and raising insulin levels.

In Conclusion

If you think sugar is a problem for you, perhaps this chapter will inspire you to get off, or at least cut back, on your sugar intake. Eliminating refined sugar and high fructose corn syrup from your diet is a big step in the right direction.

CHAPTER 14
ARTIFICIAL SWEETENERS AND HEALTHY ALTERNATIVES

Artificial sweeteners are chemicals that your body cannot break down and therefore are 100% toxic to your body.
—Dr. Lisa Vickery

Artificial sweeteners have been shown to disrupt the normal hormonal and neurological signals that control hungers and satiety (feeling of fullness). Basically, artificial sweeteners confuse your brain. The enzymes in your mouth begin a cascade that primes your cell receptors for an insulin surge and when it doesn't arrive, your brain feels cheated. In one study, people who used artificial sweeteners ate up to three times the amount of calories as the control group.

Scientists have concluded that "fake sugars" manipulate the body's natural ability to sense how much has been eaten and therefore, we overeat without realizing it. You might be asking why these toxic chemicals are allowed in our nation's food and why aren't government agencies warning us about them? A former FDA commissioner has been quoted as saying, "What the FDA is doing and what people think the FDA is doing are as different as night and day."

Artificial Sweeteners

1. **Sucrolose (Splenda)** (little yellow packet) was approved by the FDA in 1998 as a tabletop sweetener and as a general-purpose sweetener for all processed foods. Splenda is manufactured in a lab by a very complex chemical process that involves changing the structure of sugar molecules. It is created when they actually force chlorine into an unnatural bond with a sugar molecule, substituting three sucrose atoms with three chlorine atoms. While sucralose may have begun as a sugar,

it's really a synthetic chemical. One of the biggest concerns is that Splenda contains the man-made chemically-treated chlorine. "Industrial-grade chlorine is a carcinogen, any way you slice it," says toxicologist Dr. Hull. He cautions pregnant women, the elderly, and children to exercise caution with sucralose. Research suggests it may cause problems for diabetics as well.

Splenda is found in more than 4,000 packaged foods and beverages, which grabs more than 50% of the $1 billion U.S. artificial sweetener market. Dr. Joseph Mercola, author of *Sweet Deception*, cautions that Splenda has been responsible for the following symptoms: stomach cramps, flulike aches, joint pains, diarrhea, depression, migraines, dizziness, blurred vision, anxiety, blood sugar increases, and weight gain.

James Turner, chairman of the National Consumer Education group Citizens for Health, reveals the findings from scientists outlining the dangers of Splenda. In animals examined for the study, Splenda reduced the amount of good bacteria in the intestines by 50% and increased body weight. Turner states, "Splenda poses a threat to people who consume it," and verifies "the little yellow packet should carry a big red warning label."

Many people are already deficient in healthy bacteria due to consuming highly processed foods. A healthy balance of micro-organisms is required to support general health. This finding alone is reason to just say no to Splenda!

2. **Aspartame (Equal, NutraSweet, AminoSweet)** (little blue packets). Over twenty-five years ago, aspartame was first introduced into the European food supply. Despite the evidence gained over the years showing that aspartame is a dangerous toxin, it has remained on the global market with the exception of a few countries that have banned it. In fact, it continued to gain approval for use in new types of food despite evidence showing that it causes neurological brain damage, cancerous tumors, and endocrine disruption, among other things.

Today, it is an everyday component of many diet beverages, sugar-free desserts, and sugar-free chewing gums in countries worldwide. But the tides have been turning as the general public is waking up to the truth about artificial sweeteners like aspartame and the harm they cause to health. In response to the growing awareness about the dangers of artificial sweeteners, Ajinomoto, maker of aspartame, rebranded their version of aspartame, and now call it "AminoSweet" in an effort to persuade the public into accepting the chemical sweetener as natural and safe, despite evidence to the contrary.

Aspartame has had the most complaints of any food additive available to the public. It has been linked with MS, lupus, fibromyalgia, and central nervous disorders. Side effects include: migraines, panic attacks, dizziness, irritability, nausea, intestinal discomfort, skin rash, and nervousness. Some researchers have linked aspartame with depression and manic episodes. It may also contribute to male infertility.

Neurosurgeon Russell L. Blaylock, MD, has spent over a decade studying the effects of both aspartame and MSG. He says formaldehyde makes aspartame "a dangerous neurotoxin which can damage the nervous system" and is a carcinogen for many.

3. **Saccharin.** (little pink packet). Saccharin was the first widely available chemical sweetener. Better-tasting NutraSweet/Equal took its place in almost every diet soda. Most researchers agree that in sufficient doses, saccharin is carcinogenic in humans. The question is: how much artificial sweetener can your body tolerate? While saccharin appears to have fewer problems than aspartame, artificial sweeteners are body toxins. They are never a good idea to be consumed by pregnant women, children, or teenagers—despite the reduced sugar content—because of possible irreversible cell damage.

My Artificial Sugar Story—Angie L.

I was in my late twenties when I made the connection that sugar increased pain and inflammation in my body. So I quickly made the transition from sugar to artificial sugar, thinking that was a better choice for me. I drank loads of Diet Coke and used saccharin and eventually NutraSweet (Equal) and Splenda to sweeten everything. I started buying sugar-free cookies, ice cream, and candies, too. I went from one bad habit to another. When frozen yogurt stores began to offer sugar-free flavors, I was in heaven because it tasted so decadent and delicious. I sweetened my coffee, tea, and cereals with one or two pink (Saccharin), yellow (Splenda), or blue (Equal) packets.

Giving up artificial sweeteners was actually more difficult for me than giving up sugar. The reason was because I didn't noticeably react to artificial sweeteners with pain and inflammation the way I did sugar. It may have weakened me for a while on a subtle level, but not enough for me to stop.

Once at a chiropractor's (who practiced applied kinesiology) I took a sugar-free frozen yogurt that was artificially sweetened into my session to muscle test out of curiosity. Sure enough, while holding the yogurt next to my body and holding my arm out to test my strength, my arm immediately went weak. That was my body saying, "No thanks." He said, "Throw that stuff in the garbage" and tossed it into the trash. I was surprised, but not surprised. There was a part of me that knew artificial sweeteners are, well, artificial, which means unnatural, which means created with chemicals in a lab so not really good for me.

If something weakened me, I wanted to understand why. So I took the time to learn more about artificial sweeteners. As I learned more, I knew I wanted to give them up, too. This realization helped me give up Diet Coke (that was a big one for me) and all those sugar-free cookies, candies, even mints, and all those colorful packets of artificial sweeteners. It wasn't until I discovered the healthy sugar substitute, Stevia five years ago, that I was totally able to give up artificial sweeteners.

Every now and then, I will indulge in a sugar-free frozen yogurt at a yogurt shop as a special treat. Because I pay attention, I notice my energy level drops afterward. Still, I love the creamy, sweet taste. I really enjoy it while I'm eating it instead of feeling guilty. Deep down, though, I know I'm better off without it. I am very grateful for healthy sweeteners like Stevia. Sodas have hit the market that are Stevia-sweetened. I don't buy them because I prefer to make herbal tea and sweeten it myself if I want a sweet treat. But it's great to know there are healthier sweeteners than artificial sweeteners now available. Sugar substitutes don't have to be artificial. There is another way! ◆

Healthy Sugar Alternatives

The good news is that there are healthy alternatives to sugar and artificial sweeteners:

1. **Stevia** is an all-natural alternative to white sugar that's thirty times sweeter, has zero calories, zero carbs, is zero on the glycemic index, and does not raise insulin or blood sugar levels. It is our personal favorite for its taste and health benefits without the side effects.

Also known as Rebiana or Reb A., Stevia is an herb from the rainforests of the

Amazon that has been used for centuries by South Americans for 1500 years and in Japan for forty years. Since the 1970s, the Japanese have conducted extensive research on Stevia and have found it to be completely safe. In Japan, 40% of the sweetener market is Stevia-based and it's becoming more accepted worldwide.

The extract from Stevia leaves is said to be thirty times sweeter than white sugar and can be used in cooking and baking. Dr. Daniel Mowrey, who holds a doctorate in phytopharmacology and has studied Stevia extensively, states, "Few substances have ever yielded such consistently negative results in toxicity trials as have Stevia. Almost every toxicity test imaginable has been performed on Stevia extract. The results are always negative."

Stevia has significant health benefits such as improved glucose absorption, regulation of cholesterol and triglycerides, and balancing of blood sugar. It's not a surprise that Stevia is being used for treating type 2 diabetes to balance blood sugar. Stevia is available in powder or liquid form at most food stores. I like Sweet Leaf liquid brand in a bottle. When you have a sweet craving, Stevia is a safe and effective option to satisfy your sweet tooth without all of the side effects and consequences of sugar.

2. **Lo Han Kuo** (also spelled Lo Han Guo) is cultivated in the mountains of southern China. Like Stevia, lo han kuo has a natural sweet taste and contains no sugar or calories. It is a great sweetener choice for

diabetics and it also helps control food and sugar cravings. It can be found in liquid or powder form.

3. **Coconut Sugar** is produced from the sweet juices of tropical coconut palm sugar blossoms. This pure sugar alternative is naturally lower than sugar on the glycemic index (GI), which has benefits for weight control and improving glucose and lipid levels in people with diabetes (type 1 and type 2). Coconut sugar is especially high in potassium, magnesium, zinc, and iron and is a natural source of the vitamins B1, B2, B3, B6 and C. Coconut sugar is an unprocessed, unfiltered, and unbleached natural sweetener, and contains no preservatives.

4. **Other Sweeteners** such as organic honey, pure maple syrup, and agave nectar are considered healthier sweeteners than refined sugar or high fructose corn syrup but they still rank high in calories and high in sugar. Although sweeteners like molasses, fructose, and lactose are considered more "natural" and less processed, they are still high in sugar and high on the glycemic index. High glycemic index foods break down rapidly and spike blood sugar levels.

5. ***Truvia** (jointly developed by Coca-Cola and a business giant Cargill) is a combination of Stevia and Erythritol. It comes in individual powder packets and is now sold at most grocery stores.

6. ***PureVia** (jointly developed by Pepsi Co. with artificial sweetener company Merisant). While PureVia and Truvia contain mostly the same chemical formula (a combination of Stevia and Erythritol), PureVia also contains another sweetener called isomaltulose. Isomaltulose is derived from beet cane juice.

*Remember: Erythritol is a sugar alcohol, which may cause gas or bloating in some individuals.

If you have a habit of reaching for a soda when you get thirsty, you may not know there are healthier options. You may think you're not causing any health damage by ingesting artificial sweeteners, but there are health risks to be considered. If you're hooked on diet soda or sweetening your tea or coffee with artificial sweeteners, know that it's possible to change your habits with a little bit of effort. Instead of reaching for a pink, yellow, or blue packet, try one of the alternative healthy sweet options we've discussed in this chapter.

Skip the Soda: Enjoy Something Real

1. Water with cut fruit (watermelon, strawberry, raspberry, kiwi, or lime)
2. Sparkling or tonic water with juice
3. Water with lemon and Stevia (lemonade)
4. Iced herbal tea
5. Green tea
6. Coconut water
7. Carrot or other vegetable juices
8. Flavored water brands without artificial sweeteners on the market.
9. Cucumber slices, fresh ginger and mint in water
10. Nut and seed milks such as almond, hemp, or coconut milk

Below is a list that highlights the many popular forms of sugar today with our recommendation on which sugars we consider the most healthy.

Sugar Alternatives We Recommend

Brown rice syrup, date sugar, fructose from fruit, lo han kuo, organic honey, Stevia, Truvia (Stevia and Erythritol combined), vanilla extract, cinnamon

Sugar Alcohols: (low sugar/low Glycemic Index): Erythritol, isolmalt, lactitol, maltitol (avoid), mannitol, polyglycitol syrup, sorbitol (avoid), xylitol. **Note:** Sugar alcohols may cause gas and bloating in some people. Sorbitol causes the most complaints.

Less refined sugars (still high sugar/high glycemic index): Agave nectar, coconut sugar, fruit juice concentrate, honey, molasses, pure maple syrup, Sucanat

Refined (highly processed) Sugars to Avoid: White sugar, brown sugar, dextrose, cane juice, corn starch, corn sugar, high fructose corn syrup (HFCS), invert sugar, refined maple syrup, raw sugar (brown packet), turbinado sugar ("Sugar in the Raw"), sucrose

Artificial Sugars to Avoid: Aspartame (Equal, NutraSweet, AminoSweet)—blue packet, Saccharin—pink packet, Sucralose (Splenda)—yellow packet

Artificial Sweetener Facts

1. People who used artificial sweeteners eat up to three times the amount of calories as control groups.

2. Artificial sweeteners disrupt the normal hormonal and neurological signals that control hungers and satiety (feeling of fullness).

3. Artificial sweeteners confuse your brain when enzymes in your mouth prime cell receptors for an insulin surge; when it doesn't arrive your brain feels cheated.

4. Splenda (sucralose) is created when chlorine is forced into an unnatural bond with a sugar molecule, substituting three sucrose atoms with three chlorine atoms.

5. Splenda reduces the amount of good bacteria in the intestines by 50% and increases body weight.

6. Aspartame is a neurotoxin which can damage the nervous system.

7. Aspartame is responsible for the most serious complaints of any food additive available to the public.

8. While saccharin appears to have fewer problems than aspartame, artificial sweeteners are body toxins.

In Conclusion

Artificial sugars weaken the immune system and contribute to inflammation and chronic disease. While still being sold everywhere, the pink (Saccharin), yellow (Splenda), or blue (Equal) packets are artificial sweeteners that can be risky to your health. We recommend experimenting with healthier sugar alternatives listed above.

Chapter 15
Inflammation and Chronic Disease

Inflammation plays a causative role in heart disease,
Alzheimer's and Parkinson's diseases, as well as
other age-related disorders, including cancer.
—Andrew Weil, MD

What makes a normal process go out of control and why do we have an epidemic of chronic inflammatory diseases? First, we have to look at how the average person's diet has changed over the past two or three generations. Today, because of extensive food processing, our diet has become seriously out of balance. Highly-processed foods contain at least thirty times more pro-inflammatory nutrients than just 100 years ago. As a result, people have become nutritionally and biochemically primed for powerful, out-of-control, inflammatory reactions and all the diseases that accompany inflammation.

Inflammation has always played a role in infections and in healing an injured body. We need inflammation to heal. We want white blood cells rushing to the site of an injury, which produces the swelling that's part of the healing response. Then, when the job is done, inflammation and other symptoms go away. But when it becomes prolonged and gets out of control, problems begin causing damage to tissue and organs.

Many of the hidden dangers in foods set the stage for inflammation, make aches and pains worse, and increase the long-term risk of debilitating and life-threatening diseases.

The most common scenario is that once pain or inflammation sets in, our first instinct is to reach for an aspirin, ibuprofen (Advil, Motrin, Aleve) or another popular over-the-counter non-steroidal anti-inflammatory drug (NSAIDs). These are very effective in relieving headaches, controlling inflammation, easing pain, and reducing fevers. The danger is, if taken regularly, they can lead to stomach erosion (inflammation of the stomach wall) and the formation of gastric ulcers. Another mind-boggling feature of regular NSAIDS is that some of these drugs have been shown to accelerate breakdown of cartilage in joints. It is an irony that the use of NSAIDS to relieve pain can actually speed up the underlying disease process!

Reversing Mom's Chronic Disease and Inflammation —Rella H.

My mom, Chris, at seventy-six years old, started having excruciating muscle pain in her late sixties. This consisted of shooting pain in her arms and legs. The doctors had no idea what the problem was. They ran numerous tests but she continued to get worse and could hardly get out of bed. They put her on prednisone.

Initially, the prednisone worked but then the pain came back and they kept increasing her doses of prednisone. The doctor said she had "immune system deficiency" . . . that's where the immune system collapses.

They referred her to a rheumatologist who insisted it was arthritis. But I knew it wasn't in her joints but in her muscles. The doctor said her condition was "irreversible." There was nothing they could do except keep her on prednisone and that "she would not recover from this."

Out of desperation I looked for other ways to help my mom. I signed my mom and I up for Angie and Sheri's Conscious Eating class series. It was my first introduction to "Food as Medicine." Never before had I made the connection that food could heal the body.

I hadn't previously thought much about diet to help my mom with her health issues. I had assumed she was eating pretty well. She lived alone, and after looking closer at her diet, I realized it mainly consisted of fruit and cereal and very little vegetables. It was not a balanced diet.

In Sheri and Angie's Conscious Eating class, they demonstrated how to make a healthy green drink with organic vegetables and a slice of organic apple for sweetening. So at home, I started making green drinks for both of us. I put in kale, chard, spinach, blueberries, chia seeds, and flaxseeds. My mom and I each drank twelve ounces twice a day—in the morning and at dinnertime as a meal replacement. We ate a regular lunch.

Within six weeks, her immune system kicked back in, despite the doctor's prediction. (The doctor never mentioned that diet might help.) Her digestion improved. Her pain was reduced. She got stronger. She had less anxiety. Her blood sugar came into balance. Her immune system was being fed again.

What I noticed for myself was increased energy, better regularity, more clarity, and I felt less stressed.

As Mom was getting great results with the green drink, she also started seeing a doctor who practiced holistic endocrinology who put her on high doses of fish oil (1250 mg. a day) and vitamin D as a supplement. Within a year and a half, my mom was completely pain–free.

To this day, we continue making the green drinks. We add a protein powder, almond milk, and cacao powder, and continue to reap the benefits.

What I learned from this experience is that the immune system is created and supported by what we eat. ♦

Jack Challem, in his book, *The Inflammation Syndrome*, describes a new way of viewing inflammation disorders as a consequence of eating an unbalanced diet. He states that "Foods like white bread, pastries, white rice, and refined sugars have the effect of turbo–charging our inflammatory production pathways, while other foods have the precise opposite effect." In our experience, we found this to be true.

Inflammation and Diet: Making the Connection —Angie L.

I know that my poor eating habits largely contributed to inflammation and eventually getting arthritis. There is no history of arthritis in my family. Starting at a young age, my daily snacking largely consisted of baked goods, bread, graham crackers, candy, candy bars, and diet soda.

Later in my life, it was easy to see the direct connection between certain foods and inflammation. By changing my diet and eliminating these offending foods, in addition to focusing on high quality foods and supplements, my body came back into total balance. ◆

Physicians have long recognized inflammation as the culprit in asthma, arthritis, and many other conditions. More recently, the medical community has been redefining inflammation as the root of most chronic diseases.

Understanding what causes chronic inflammation is crucial to preventing critical health issues such as heart disease, cancer, arthritis, Alzheimer's, diabetes, and obesity. Chronic inflammation reduces your odds of living a long life.

Inflammation and Chronic Disease

How does chronic inflammation set the stage for chronic disease? It slowly wears down our bodies, contributing to aging and degeneration. In scientific terms, inflammation is the complex biological response to harmful stimuli, such as pathogens, damaged cells, or irritants. It is also a process by which the body's white blood cells protect our bodies from infection by foreign substances, such as bacteria and viruses. This release of chemicals leaks fluid into the tissues which stimulates nerves and causes pain—necessary for healing but when it becomes chronic, health problems begin.

Inflammation that is unregulated can result in excessive free radical activity and tissue destruction. Although free radicals perform some beneficial functions within the immune system, scientists believe they do much more harm than good. If there are too many free radicals, or they exist in the wrong places, they can attack and damage healthy cells. Free radicals have been linked to aging, tissue damage, rheumatoid arthritis, diabetes, cardiovascular disease, and some types of cancer.

Another key scenario that sets the stage for inflammation is high levels of glucose (sugar). This starts a chain reaction that produces large amounts of free radicals that stimulates inflammatory responses and high levels of inflammation. This increases the risk of many diseases.

My Experience with Inflammation—Sheri M.

My history of Lyme disease and ulcerative colitis (inflammation of the intestinal tract) involved both pain and inflammation. Although my gastroenterologist (gut doctor) prescribed anti-inflammatory drugs, he offered no dietary advice.

By doing my own research and working with a naturopathic doctor, I began to manage these conditions. I practiced stress reduction through yoga and meditation and learned about the anti-inflammation diet. The first step I took was eliminating wheat and within a month I was wheat- and gluten-free. In addition, I followed a low-carb, low-sugar diet and the inflammatory symptoms of intestinal discomfort and joint pain soon diminished. My ulcerative colitis was in remission within a couple of months. ♦

Anti-Inflammation Diet Tips
- Eat a variety of fresh, whole foods.
- Whenever possible, buy and eat organically–raised foods.
- Minimize eating processed foods and eliminate fast foods. Focus 80% of your diet on alkaline foods.
- For omega-3 fatty acids, eat more wild fish, especially cold-water varieties like wild salmon, sardines, herring, and black cod; hemp seeds and flax oil; fish oil; cod liver oil; and flaxseeds, preferably fresh ground.

- Eat grass-fed (not corn fed) lean organic meats from free-range chicken, turkey, and game meats such as duck and pheasant.
- Eat an abundance of antioxidant-containing foods like broccoli, kale, strawberries, spinach, brussel sprouts, melons and cabbages.
- Eat carotene-containing foods like sweet potatoes, carrots, squash, and pumpkin.
- Eat a moderate amount of fruit, the more colorful the better.
- Use spices and herbs such as turmeric and ginger to flavor foods.
- Use cold–pressed extra virgin olive oil to drizzle on salads or cooked vegetables. Use coconut oil or butter for heating at high temperatures.
- Eat sprouted gluten-free grains such as brown or wild rice, quinoa, millet, buckwheat, or gluten-free oats.
- Snack on nuts (except peanuts), cashews (in small quantities), almonds, sunflower seeds, and pumpkin seeds.
- Drink clean, filtered water and herbal, non-caffeinated teas with or without stevia.
- Drink rice, hemp, almond, coconut, or goat milk instead of cow milk.

Avoid the Following Pro-Inflammatory Foods

- White, bleached, refined flour or products made from these processed foods.
- Refined sugar, raw sugar, brown sugar, molasses, high fructose corn syrup, or products made with these such as jams, ice cream, pastries, cookies, and candies.
- Milk or cream (very small amounts of cow's milk allowed)
- Fried foods
- Canned (tinned) foods
- Alcoholic beverages
- Cooking oils such as corn, soybean, and canola, mixed vegetable oils as well as vegetable shortening, margarine and partial–hydrogenated oils.
- Identify and avoid food allergens. The eight most common are: wheat (gluten), dairy, sugar, corn, soy, MSG, yeast, and alcohol.

Nightshades are also an issue for some people. Most common are potatoes, tomatoes, and peppers.

- Refined and highly–processed carbohydrates (i.e. junk food)
- Unfiltered tap water
- Soft drinks (regular and diet)
- Artificial sweeteners (Splenda, sucralose, aspartame, NutraSweet, Equal)
- All foods containing artificial flavorings, additives, and preservatives
- Omega-6 fatty acids (margarine, shortening, and hydrogenated oils are super inflammatory they are found in baked goods, ice cream, chocolate, candy, potato chips, and packaged foods.)

More Inflammation Facts

- Inflammation plays a causative role in heart disease, Alzheimer's, Parkinson's disease, and cancer as well as other disorders.
- Elevated inflammation levels increase the risk of a heart attack by four and a half times.
- High glucose levels set the stage for inflammation.
- Because of extensive food processing, our diet has become seriously unbalanced.
- Highly processed foods contain at least thirty times more pro-inflammatory nutrients than just 100 years ago.
- Omega-3 lubricates joints and lines the digestive tract to help prevent the entrance of foreign material.

In Conclusion

Inflammation can be triggered by many factors such as diet, stress, physical injuries, infections, and environmental stressors (air pollution, allergies to pollen, mold, chemicals in food and water). The factor that we have the most control over is our diet. Focus your diet on foods that are natural inflammation fighters to reduce all forms of inflammation in your body.

CHAPTER 16
ACID ALKALINE,
CANDIDA, AND ENZYMES

Most diseases originate from an acid state.

Acidosis is a condition of over-acidity in the blood and body tissues. In the body, acid converts to mucous. Mucous converts to inflammation. Inflammation converts to disease. When the body loses its alkaline reserve, virus, bacteria, yeast, and fungus take over and can cause degenerative diseases such as diabetes, cancer, AIDS, arteriosclerosis, arthritis, osteoporosis, chronic fatigue, and the list goes on.

Causes of acidosis may include: improper diet, kidney, liver and adrenal disorders, emotional disturbances, fever, an excess of niacin, and aspirin. Chemicals create cell mutations which change the pH in the body. Industrial pollution, harmful chemicals in foods and in the ground also increase the acidity of our pH. Patricia's story illustrates how alkalizing one's diet can result in increased energy, weight loss, and even improved eyesight.

How My Life Improved with an Alkaline Diet
—Patricia A.

Before I changed my way of eating, I was always sick with a cold or allergies, my eyes and skin had a yellowish appearance, and my eyesight was deteriorating. I thought my decrease in energy was due to getting older. When my eye prescription had to be changed frequently, I knew I had to do something. After doing some research on diet, I decided to reduce the acidic foods in my diet and add more alkalizing foods.

I had not been including many vegetables in my diet and would eat what I now realize was 80% acid foods. For breakfast I'd have white toast and jelly with fried eggs and thought I was eating well. I had little energy throughout the day.

To change my diet, I began having smoothies for breakfast which included protein powder; rice, almond, or hempseed milk; and green vegetables such as kale or spinach, or green vegetable powder. Sometimes I use vegetable juice. Just changing my breakfast gave me so much more energy.

For lunch I often have vegetable soup or tempeh (fermented tofu), a big salad, and almond butter on celery or whole grain crackers.

I eat a lot of salads using many different vegetables and always top it with avocado, my favorite treat. I snack on nuts, celery, carrots, slices of cucumber, sometimes dipping them in hummus or salsa. Almond butter and apple slices are like having a dessert for me. I eliminated sugar and no longer have sugar cravings.

I often make stir fries for dinner, using broccoli or kale, and sometimes I add a small amount of fish or chicken. I eat beans, lentils with a little brown rice and vegetables, and a nice big salad. I use lemon juice and olive oil on my salads.

I also have cut down on my dairy intake and just have goat yogurt or kefir now and then.

My diet has gone from mostly acid forming foods to 80% alkalizing foods. As a result, I am healthier than I've ever been and no longer get colds and the flu and my allergies disappeared.

I have gradually gained more energy and vitality. I need less sleep and don't need to take naps anymore because of sustained energy throughout the day. My eyesight has improved and I lost thirty-five pounds. This new way of eating has made a total difference for me and I am encouraging my friends to change to a more alkaline diet. I want to feel good so I plan to continue eating this way for the rest of my life. ♦

Optimum pH Levels

When the body produces excess acid, it's dumped into the tissues for storage. The lymphatic system neutralizes it as best as it can and gets rid of excess acid by dumping it back into the bloodstream. The imbalance in the blood pH leads to inflammation and sets the stage for disease. Blood is the most accurate test for pH, then urine, then saliva.

Microforms thrive in an acidic environment. Microforms are yeast, fungus, mold, bacteria, and viruses whose waste is poisonous and toxic. Their waste products further pollute our system. Excess acidity results in low oxygen which microforms love. These toxins reduce the absorption of protein, minerals, and other nutrients, which weakens the body's ability to produce enzymes and the hundreds of other chemical components necessary for cell and organ activity.

Microforms are major players in chronic fatigue syndrome. An overly acidic environment contributes to excess weight gain. In a defensive maneuver, the body creates fat cells to carry acids away from your vital organs to try to protect them. But when you reduce the acid load, your body won't need to keep the fat around anymore. Their leftover toxins can be bound up by certain fats and minerals and eliminated from the body. The optimum pH for our blood and body tissues is about 7.2. Alkaline refers to a substance or solution that has a pH of 7.0 or above. Saliva and urine tests from a healthy body should be about 6.6 to 6.8. The body heals best when it is slightly alkaline. To keep the blood and body tissue at an optimum pH, limit acid-forming food. Make sure your food intake is 80% alkaline and drink plenty of clean, filtered water.

How to Test—Sheri M.

I use saliva pH test strips from time to time to be sure I'm in the normal pH range. When I'm too acidic, I feel tired and heavy, especially in the morning. Overall, I just don't feel my best. That's when I know I need to focus on alkalizing foods, mainly leafy green vegetables, pumpkin seeds, flaxseeds, legumes, wild rice, herbal teas, and filtered water. And I avoid sugar which is highly acid forming. ♦

Candida, the Yeasty Beasties

Millions of Americans, most without even realizing it, suffer from candida, a yeast overgrowth. Candida compromises the immune system and is primarily caused by diets high in sugars and starches, medications, birth control pills, alcohol, chemotherapy, chemicals and toxins, diabetes, excessive stress, having a repressed immune system, chronic constipation or diarrhea, intestinal parasites, and food allergies that inflame the colon.

Mood Swings, Depression, Brain Fog, Headaches, and Fatigue: My Candida Story—Sarah C.

It was an icy winter afternoon in late December when I dragged myself home from school and collapsed onto my bed, overwhelmed with exhaustion.

I was pulled into darkness in a matter of seconds as the fatigue that struggled to overtake me all day finally won.

It felt as if there was constantly something wrong with me, and I had no way to escape it.

I was dominated by these feelings every minute of the day, and soon it didn't seem like I was living a normal life anymore.

I was overly tired all the time, had mood swings, was depressed, had brain fog and headaches which caused me to do badly in school, and I was allergic to almost everything.

I suffered from a chronic yeast infection called candida for eight years before I finally discovered what it was that was wrong with me for most of my life.

Candida feeds on yeast, which includes any foods with sugar or wheat. To starve the candida, I had to stay away from these foods.

Cutting out sugar and wheat (gluten) was a challenge at first, but the effects were so prominent and so incredible that it was worth it. If I had kept eating the way I did, I would have been severely ill by the time I was twenty. Just as important, I would never have been able to enjoy life.

It has now been four years since I've been diagnosed with candida, and my life has completely changed. I was able to heal simply through natural medicine and by changing my diet. ◆

Candida (yeast) exists in balance with normal intestinal flora and is necessary for digestion, absorbing nutrition, and preventing infection. However, when this yeast becomes overgrown, it can overtake normal, friendly, beneficial bacteria. Many factors lead to this overgrowth.

Common expressions of candida overgrowth include vaginal yeast infections, thrush (a white yeast infection of the mouth), dandruff, itchy skin, headaches, depression, mood swings, intense food cravings for sweet and starchy foods (yeast's best food source), and fatigue. Candida can colonize in the intestinal tract and migrate to other parts and organs of the body. The presence of candida in the intestines can cause reactions like bloating and inflammation.

Consuming yeast in the diet, from bread to wine and beer can aggravate these symptoms or cause additional allergic reactions.

If you suspect you have candida, your best defense is to starve the candida that lives mainly on all forms of sugar.

To starve the candida, one must eliminate sugar, alcohol, fruit, and grains for sixty to ninety days. Taking a high-quality probiotic daily (such as Reuteri or Culturelle) speeds healing time. The best way to take a probiotic is first thing upon waking on an empty stomach. In addition, take digestive enzymes with every meal. Some studies suggest that candida overgrowth results from an enzyme imbalance in the digestive tract.

Candida (yeast) exists in balance with normal intestinal flora and is necessary for digestion, absorbing nutrition, and preventing infection. However, when this yeast becomes overgrown, it can overtake normal, friendly, beneficial bacteria. Maintaining an alkaline state in the blood and body helps slow the overgrowth of candida in addition to following an anti-candida diet.

Probiotics and Enzymes

There are easy preventative measures we can take to safeguard our health. Two such measures are supplementing with probiotics and digestive enzymes. The World Health Organization refers to probiotics as live microorganisms that provide essential health benefits.

Probiotics are referred to as "friendly" bacteria responsible for several important biological functions. Some of these functions include assisting with digestion, keeping other harmful bacteria at bay and stimulating the immune system.

Here's a story where one mother discovers the power of probiotics to heal her son's condition.

Discovering the Power of Probiotics—Erica O.

In the spring of 2013, our four-year-old son started having diarrhea. The issue did not resolve itself after a week, so we took him to the doctor. Our pediatrician had retired, so we were consulting with the assigned replacement in the large HMO. Turned out the replacement was the head of pediatrics at that facility. We felt confident, then, that the prescribed "take some Activia every day and feed him the BRAT diet" would heal him in no time. The BRAT diet, prescribed for gastrointestinal distress, is bland and low in insoluble fiber (bananas, rice, applesauce, and toast). Our son, who didn't like to eat bananas, rice, or toast, was challenging to feed. He was used to a high fiber fruit and vegetable diet intermixed with healthy fish and meats as well as grain products. We fed him the Activia every day, even though the sugar grams were high. The pediatrician claimed that the live cultures would be beneficial although the 'sugars' were technically not part of the recommended diet. And we fed what our son would eat. By week three, he still had diarrhea and now was quite lethargic, not wanting to get off the couch and run around at the park like he used to. Then we headed off on vacation for a week, with continued diarrhea and lethargy. By week five, he had lost four pounds from his forty-two-pound body. We made another appointment with the head of pediatrics.

In the meantime, we purchased some Culturelle for Kids as recommended by Angie. She stated that the Activia did not have sufficient cultures to turn around our son's issues. It was in this four-day window before our next appointment that we saw a real turn-around for our son. The diarrhea was already resolving and energy was coming back to our boy! We still went to the appointment and told the head of pediatrics of this turn-around. We expressed that the probiotic had 10 billion lactobacillus cells in each daily child's chew versus the small amount in the recommended yogurt.

This large HMO could only spit out what was recommended from the computer system. We tried to educate her and the program with our real-life experiment. We simply stated that the Culturelle is the only reason our son gained back his weight and energy.

We are entirely grateful to those who understand the perspective of natural healing outside of Western medicine. We spread the word of these chewable probiotics to other parents of young children often. It shouldn't have taken so long to heal our child. Now we know. ♦

Erica's story proves that a simple, quality probiotic can heal a gut issue. Physicians in Europe routinely prescribe potent probiotics to treat chronic disease. The problem is that many U.S. doctors overprescribe antibiotics which kill not only the bad bacteria but also the good bacteria.

Many of the foods being marketed as probiotics contain little or no health value, according to researchers. Supplementing with a quality probiotic is very important if you suspect you have gut-related issues such as dysbiosis, candida, or leaky gut.

Enzymes

Enzymes are the work horses for maintaining a healthy body. They build strong bones and nerve tissue, and attack cancerous cells and carry them out of the body. They also clean up the blood and tissue, dissolve foreign substances, and slow the aging process by maintaining the body's health at the cellular level.

In fact, the entire cycle of life is dependent on enzyme activity. They are so important in our health and well-being, that not even vitamins, minerals, or hormones have any value without them.

Dr. Edward Howell, a pioneer in enzyme research, is formally recognized as having discovered the vital role of enzymes in human nutrition. Howell states, "The increased use of food enzymes promotes a decreased rate of exhaustion of the enzyme potential." In other words, supplementing with enzymes keeps enzyme levels from decreasing.

Tests have shown that a seventy-year-old person has only about half the enzyme level of a twenty-year-old. A newborn baby has 100 times the enzymes levels of an elderly person. As we become enzyme-deficient, we age faster.

When enzyme levels are low, food cannot be properly broken down and digested. The intestinal track becomes congested with partially digested food that makes the intestinal tract resemble a clogged sewer pipe. Undigested food particles cling to intestines forming walls of encrustation that block vitamins and minerals from being absorbed by the body. Subsequently, food contents lodged in the intestinal track putrefy and turn toxic. Bacteria and parasites begin to flourish and live in the bowel. Eventually, this condition creates holes in the lining of the intestine allowing partially digested food particles, toxins, bacteria, and parasites to seep through the bowel wall and into the bloodstream. Because enzyme action is missing in the digestive tract to eliminate this condition, the body has no way of destroying this toxic brew.

The condition that results is leaky gut syndrome. You will learn more about this in the chapter Leaky Gut Syndrome.

There are three types of enzymes:

1. **Metabolic enzymes** help our cells detox and produce energy.

2. **Digestive enzymes** break down our food into nutrients and waste.

3. **Food enzymes** are obtained through the raw foods we eat; cooking and heating over 115 degrees destroys food enzymes.

Many people would benefit from taking a digestive enzyme with the largest meal of the day to better process and absorb nutrients. Consult your health practitioner to determine the enzyme that's best for you.

Digestive enzyme supplements can contain the following:

1. **Protease** digests protein.

2. **Lipase** digests fat.

3. **Amylase** digests carbs.

4. **Cellulase** breaks down fiber.

5. **Invertase** digests sugars.

6. **Lactase** digests lactose (dairy sugar).

7. **Diatase** digests starches and sugars.

In Conclusion

Acidosis is a condition of over-acidity in the blood and body tissues. Alkalizing one's diet can result in increased energy, weight loss, and even improved eyesight.

Probiotics are "good" bacteria that restore balance to the microflora-bacteria that live in the intestines. A quality probiotic can often help heal a gut-related issue.

Many people would benefit from taking a digestive enzyme with the largest meal of the day to better process and absorb nutrients. Consult your health practitioner or nutritionist to determine the supplement that's best for you.

Chapter 17
Arthritis

The best way out is always through.
—Robert Frost

When we hear the term arthritis, we usually think of cracking joints and stiffness in the morning. There are more than 100 conditions that are identified as arthritis. The two major forms are rheumatoid arthritis (RA) and osteoarthritis (OA). More than 22% of American adults (50 million) have arthritis. As baby boomers grow older and people live longer in general, that number is expected to double.

Rheumatoid Arthritis

Rheumatoid arthritis (RA) is a systemic disease of altered immunity—an autoimmune disease—affecting not only the joints but also the eyes, muscles, nerves, and other organs. With RA, the body attacks its own tissues as a result of a faulty immune system reaction.

While this condition most commonly develops in people between the ages of twenty-five and fifty, it can occur at any age. It can cause crippling and deformity of joints at an early age, including in children. Women are affected three times more than men.

If you have been struggling with arthritis, know that many people have been able to reverse symptoms by changing their diet!

My Experience with Arthritis—Angie L.

I was diagnosed with rheumatoid arthritis when I was in college at age twenty. I had severe pain all over my body, especially my joints, making it difficult to walk or even get out of bed in the morning. After a decade of taking the recommended prescription arthritis drugs including cortisone shots and surgeries, I was inspired to look at my diet and make necessary changes. I began by eliminating gluten, dairy, and sugar, and started taking glucosamine chondroitin with MSM along with a quality nutrition supplement. By being more mindful of what I was putting into my body, the pain and inflammation in my body dramatically lessened within weeks. Within a year, I was pain-free and drug-free and no longer needed these supplements.

My personal experience validates that rheumatoid arthritis can be reversed with proper diet, quality supplements, and a belief that it is possible. ♦

Rachna's compelling story below further illustrates that the symptoms of RA can be reversed or dramatically reduced by following an anti-inflammatory diet. Like Angie, Rachna had such an advanced case of RA she, too, was put on the chemotherapy drug, Methotrexate.

How I Became the Change—Rachna C.

Just because you're not sick doesn't mean you're healthy.

Thirteen steroid injections jabbed into my bones: my knuckles, wrists, two of my fingers, one elbow, and one thumb. My left thumb was so swollen that despite trying to shove the needle in thrice, the needle wouldn't go in, so the rheumatologist gave up.

I sat up on the bed, remembering this as my last clear memory. My pillow was a mass of fallen hair—hair unable to withstand the onslaught of a banned chemotherapy drug called Methotrexate—which rheumatologists continue to prescribe to patients of autoimmune disorders. Hair brittled by steroids prescribed to reduce inflammation in the bones, the same steroids that ironically, in the long run, weaken the already weakened bones. All this, whirred in my head as I got off the bed, and limped into the living room.

Why such odds? Why is the treatment of an autoimmune disorder so conflicting in medical science? Isn't there a logical cure that goes to the root cause and roots it out? I asked myself all these questions.

I saw the problem as a work issue: how we resolve stumbling blocks or a slowdown or losing business. Think alternative. Think innovative. Think lateral. Think creative. I opened my laptop with my swollen fingers and started researching, reading, trying to find people similar to me who had found a less painful, more permanent solution.

I visited bookstores, ordered books online, and was immersed in some serious rheumatoid arthritis (RA) reading. A new strength was beginning to seep in, a defiance I'm very comfortable with as a person.

I was going to use the same attitude toward finding a solution to my health problem. Equipped with my knowledge, I went to my rheumatologist. Surely he would help answer some of my questions. He had treated so many patients, he had specialized in the field, he knew me.

He knew the side effects of the medications which he had told me about when I started them—that they would affect the liver and kidneys so every two months, I needed to get a blood test done to see if my liver and kidneys were okay. He and the medical community were still looking for a permanent cure to RA, and his experiences would help me find a solution.

But all he had to say was, "You will be bedridden."

I couldn't believe my ears. I had been sitting for forty-five minutes with this man, who claimed to be an RA specialist, sharing my understanding of where the root cause of RA lay, and attacking it, and all he had to say was, "You will be bedridden. And crippled."

"How can you say that?"

"Sixty-seven percent of people with your aggression of RA never go back to a normal life. If you leave your medication, you will not be able to stop the deformities and pain," he said, with the authority of God.

"But even after these medications, you have not been able to stop my finger, toes, and wrist from deformities, so how can you say that?"

"Imagine what they will be if you don't take the medicines," he said haughtily.

"Well, I don't want to make a choice. I am limping right now, not walking. I want to walk and run like I used to, and I want my hair back. So I will not take these pills that are ruining my body and my organs."

"The choice is yours. This is the treatment. If you don't follow it, you will be bedridden."

"Sure, I'm willing to take that chance." I said that, and walked out. I went straight to the restroom, and burst into tears. I sat on the pot for ten minutes and cried my heart out, lamenting the world, God, and myself; pitying myself, feeling lost, feeling hopeless, feeling like ending my life. I had taken a drastic step to not follow what the medical world knew as a cure to my disease. I had so much pain that my thirty-six-hour labor and childbirth seemed like a piece of cake in comparison.

And I had nowhere to go.

Throughout the day, my mind was whirring with pinning on to the logic of why and how this disease takes route, based on the millions of pages I had read and my own symptoms. And my first logic that came out was something like this: RA is an inflammatory disease—inflammation is internal and external—medicines and treatment suppress the inflammation. So what causes inflammation?

And hence started my journey toward curing myself.

Over the next few months, I continued the immune suppressants as the doc had prescribed them, because I knew that not taking them could leave me completely bedridden with pain. But I completely stopped Methotrexate and steroids, because I knew they were doing more harm than good. Simultaneously, I started attacking my inflammation in other ways. I had researched on what caused inflammation, and I came across "inflammatory" foods and lifestyle on the internet and in the books I read. I then came across "anti-inflammatory" foods and lifestyle. What if I eliminated inflammatory foods and replaced them with anti-inflammatory foods? Surely that would bring the inflammation down.

Hence I started the process of elimination. Out went carbohydrates, especially white flour, sugar, and processed foods. In came fresh fruits, vegetables, nuts, green tea, and red wine. I hired a yoga teacher, who worked with my swollen, slow joints, and gently pushed me three times a week, to regain my flexibility.

During my heated discussion with my rheumatologist, he had shared with me that in mild cases of RA, ayurvedic treatment had shown some improvement, but my case was too aggressive for that. Now that I had conquered two inflammation points—food and exercise—it was time to start healing and strengthening my joints as well. So I signed up for a fourteen-day massage therapy specifically designed for RA patients at a local, well–known ayurvedic center. For seven days, they "opened" up my body with abhyanga, letting the oils seep in and the gentle massage get rid of the stiffness. Then for the next seven days, they performed potli massage, where they pounded the affected joints with a small cloth bag full of herbs dipped in hot ayurvedic oil, to heal the joints. Post the fourteen days, there was a repeat of potli every twenty-one days.

I followed it religiously. A day after potli started, my pains returned very badly and my entire body couldn't move. The ayurvedic doctor said that initially in potli, the pain will return before going away. I had already suffered so much, so waiting around for twenty-four to forty-eight hours didn't seem to daunt me. And sure enough, the pains began receding after forty-eight hours. After my fourteen-day ayurvedic treatment, I did feel better. But the pain remained.

I had started my hit and miss treatment in October. By December, my pains had reduced by 80%. I was eating a sattvic diet, and had given up lentils completely since they contained proteins that flared up any pain, but had cheated with coffee.

By January, I began tapering off the immune suppressants, but my 20% pain levels remained. At that point, I decided to listen to Runvijay sir, and increased my pranayama (breath control) to ten minutes. Within a week, I felt relief. I increased it a bit more, to fifteen minutes the next week, and noticed the difference in pain. By February end, my pranayama was at thirty minutes, and my pain, at 3%. I was, for the first time since my RA, almost pain–free. And that's when I got my blood tests for RA done. And the reports were...negative. My RA had gone. ◆

Rheumatoid Arthritis Facts

- 50 million American adults have arthritis diagnosed by a doctor. Nearly two-thirds of arthritis patients are under sixty-five years old.
- By 2030, the number of people with arthritis is expected to rise to 67 million, reflecting a 40% increase.
- An estimated 294,000 children under age eighteen have some form of arthritis; this represents approximately one in every 250 children in the U.S.
- More than 60% of arthritis patients are women.
- RA can double a woman's risk of suffering a heart attack.
- Disease rates are similar for whites and African-Americans; Hispanic people have lower RA rates.
- Arthritic people can react to any food and do so according to their individual genetic blueprint.
- Many people with arthritis react to gluten.

Osteoarthritis (OA)

Osteoarthritis is the most common form of joint disease and is generally considered to be due to "wear–and–tear of the joints," which leads to damage of the joint surfaces and pain with movement. It causes pain, swelling, stiffness, and limited mobility of any given joint and is sometimes caused by an injury or defect in the protein part of cartilage. OA involves deterioration of the cartilage that covers the end of the bone.

Osteoarthritis Facts

- Osteoarthritis (OA) is the most common type of arthritis. Nearly 27 million Americans have it.

- As age increases, osteoarthritis prevalence affects the hands and knees of women more frequently than men.
- As age increases, OA affects African-Americans more frequently than whites.
- Disability results most often when OA affects the spine and weight-bearing joints (knees and hips).

Most people, as well as doctors, are of the belief that arthritis is incurable and that its symptoms can only be suppressed with drugs such as Methotrexate, Celebrex, prednisone and biologic self-injections such as Enbrel and Humira, and pill forms of these drugs with new drugs continually being developed.

The single most effective natural treatment for arthritis is diet. In addition to following the anti-inflammation diet, you can determine which food may be causing you the most inflammation and aggravation by following this elimination diet:

- Begin by eliminating gluten, sugar, or dairy.
- Give up one food at a time for two weeks and notice how you feel.
- Notice if your pain level, swelling, stiffness, and/or fatigue diminishes.
- If you notice a reduction in some of these symptoms, continue to stay off the food you eliminated.

After about a month, try adding back one food at a time and notice if your symptoms return.

Below are tips for what to eat and what to avoid eating if you have rheumatoid arthritis or osteoarthritis. Realizing that specific foods ignite the inflammatory process and avoiding those foods is the best strategy for reducing long-term disease risks.

Foods and Beverages That Help Reverse Arthritis

- Eat a variety of fresh, whole foods.
- Buy and eat organically raised foods whenever possible. Minimize eating processed foods and eliminate fast foods.

Focus your diet on alkaline reacting foods such as vegetables and some fruit.

- For omega-3 fatty acids, eat more wild fish, especially cold-water varieties like wild salmon, sardines, herring, and black cod; flax oil; fish oil; cod liver oil; hemp seeds; and flaxseeds, preferably fresh ground. Omega-3 lubricates joints and lines the digestive tract to help prevent the entrance of foreign material and are natural inflammation fighters.
- Eat grass-fed (not corn–fed) lean organic meats from free-range chicken, turkey, and game meats such as duck and pheasant.
- Eat an abundance of antioxidant-containing foods like broccoli, kale, strawberries, spinach, brussel sprouts, melons, and cabbages.
- Eat carotene-containing foods like sweet potatoes, carrots, squash, and pumpkin.
- Eat a moderate amount of fruit: the more colorful the better.
- Eat more beans, winter squashes, sweet potatoes, and avocados.
- Use spices and herbs such as turmeric and ginger to flavor foods.
- Use cold pressed extra virgin olive oil as your primary cooking oil. Coconut oil is also good and can be heated to high temperatures.
- Eat sprouted gluten-free grains such as brown or wild rice, quinoa, millet, buckwheat, or gluten–free oats.
- Snack on nuts (except peanuts) such as almonds, walnuts, pecans, and cashews in small quantities, sunflower seeds, and pumpkin seeds.
- Avoid cow dairy and drink dairy alternative milks such as rice, hemp, almond, coconut, or goat milk.
- Drink clean, filtered water and herbal teas. These can be sweetened with Stevia.

Foods and Beverages That Contribute to Arthritis Symptoms

- White, bleached, refined flour, highly processed carbohydrates, or products made from these processed foods
- Refined sugar, raw sugar, brown sugar, molasses, high fructose corn syrup, or products made with these such as jams, ice cream, pastries, cookies, and candies
- Milk or cream (very small amounts of cow's milk allowed).
- Fried foods
- Canned (tinned) foods
- Alcoholic beverages
- Cooking oils such as corn, soybean oil, and canola oils, mixed vegetable oils as well as vegetable shortening, margarine, and partially hydrogenated oils
- Unfiltered tap water
- Soft drinks (regular and diet)
- Artificial sweeteners (Splenda, sucralose, aspartame, NutraSweet, Equal)
- All foods containing artificial flavorings, additives, and preservatives
- Omega-6 Fatty Acids (margarine, shortening, and hydrogenated oils are super inflammatory and found in baked goods, ice cream, chocolate, candy, potato chips, and packaged foods.)
- Coffee. Some people can handle coffee well and even enjoy some of its health benefits, but it's not for everyone. If you have arthritis or a compromised immune system, coffee is not recommended. According to Dr. Mark Hyman, the caffeine in coffee increases catecholamines, your stress hormones. The stress response elicits cortisol and increases insulin. Insulin increases inflammation.
- Identify any avoid food allergens or sensitivities.

My Supplementation—Sheri M.

To address Lyme-related arthritis, I supplement with one capsule daily of curcumin (the yellow pigment of the herb turmeric) called "Curamin," which is a complex of herbs known for their anti-inflammatory properties. In some studies it has been reported to be as effective as cortisone without any of the associated side effects. Curcumin (turmeric) is primarily effective as a natural anti-inflammatory agent but it also has important uses in cancer prevention, liver disorders, heart disease, and irritable bowel syndrome. I also take a half teaspoon of methylsulfonylmethane (MSM) powder. ♦

Alex Goldstein, owner of Natural Life health food store in Northern California, has been an invaluable resource to me through the years. He offers generous discounts and ships products world wide. For more information, go to https://naturallifefoods.com.

MSM

MSM is a natural form of organic sulfur component that helps reduce pain and inflammation. Please note that some people may be allergic to sulfur (MSM) supplements.

A deficiency of MSM can result in fatigue and an increased susceptibility of arthritis. MSM can be taken in combination with glucosamine and chondroitin and can be purchased together in capsule form.

My Supplementation—Angie L.

In the early days of reversing arthritis and changing my diet, I supplemented with glucosamine chondroitin with MSM. Within a couple years, I was able to manage arthritis with an anti-inflammatory diet and no longer needed to take this combination supplement. ♦

Numerous double-blind studies concluded that supplementation with glucosamine sulfate also helps reverse arthritis. Glucosamine sulfate actually works to repair the damage and is an effective pain reliever as well. Glucosamine studies show it helps with joint tenderness, pain, and joint swelling. Chondroitin sulfate taken orally also appears to have a beneficial effect. When glucosamine sulfate and chondroitin sulfate are taken together, they work synergistically to stimulate cartilage production and help control enzymes that destroy cartilage. The book *The Arthritis Cure* by Jason Theodosakis, MD, emphasizes the power of the supplements glucosamine and chondroitin as a natural arthritis cure.

Testing for Arthritis

Clinical diagnosis of rheumatoid arthritis is based on symptoms, physical exam, X-rays, and blood tests. Typically, a rheumatologist (an expert in autoimmune diseases) performs the diagnosis and offers treatment options.

Rheumatoid Factor

Rheumatoid factor (RF) is commonly used as a blood test for the diagnosis of rheumatoid arthritis. RF is present in about 80% of adults (but a much lower proportion of children) with rheumatoid arthritis.

Rheumatoid factor is an antibody that is measurable in the blood and is actually an antibody that can bind to other antibodies. Antibodies are normal proteins in our blood that are important parts of our immune system. Rheumatoid factor is an antibody that is not usually present in the normal individual.

Rheumatoid factor is also present in patients with other conditions, including other connective tissue diseases (such as systemic lupus), some infectious diseases (such as infectious hepatitis, syphilis, infectious mononucleosis, parasites, and tuberculosis), liver disease, and sarcoidosis. Rheumatoid factor can also sometimes be present in normal individuals without diseases. This occurs more frequently in people with family members who have rheumatoid arthritis.

In Conclusion

Ask yourself these questions: Am I taking anti-inflammatory pills to alleviate pain and inflammation? Do I experience: Stiffness in the morning? Stiffness after sitting in one position? Pain in my joints? Swelling in hands, feet, or other joints? Limited mobility?

A good place to start is to remove all forms of refined white (and brown) sugar, wheat and white flour (gluten) from your diet. Consult with your doctor to confirm a diagnosis. Know that your medical doctor may or may not discuss diet with you so consider seeing a nutritionist or integrative physician. We believe strongly that you can completely cure yourself of arthritis and inflammation with discipline by following an anti-inflammatory diet.

CHAPTER 18
HEALTHY BRAIN, HAPPY YOU

You can absolutely do things early on in life and throughout your lifetime that work to maintain the bulk and function of the brain.
—Dr. David Perlmutter, author of *Power Up Your Brain*

Did you know that your brain has more connections in it than there are stars in the universe? Your brain and nervous system are the most important and complex parts of your body. They regulate your internal body functions and coordinate your responses to the outside environment. Your brain is the seat of your intelligence, memory, will, and emotion. It is the command and control center running your life and is involved in absolutely everything you do. It determines how you think, act and how well you get along with other people.

During the past twenty years, advanced imaging techniques and chemical studies of brain cells have improved our understanding of brain function dramatically. The underlying mechanism allowing these changes to occur is a unique quality known as neuroplasticity: the ability of the human brain to structurally rearrange itself in response to a wide variety of positive and negative events. Rather than seeing the brain as an organ that slowly matures during the first two decades of life, then withers away as we age, scientists now look at the human brain as a constantly changing mass of activity. *It is never too late to improve your brain.*

Food and the Brain

"All aspects of diet can affect all aspects of psychological and emotional functioning, and the fact that the average doctor sees no connection between nutrition and the mind is staggering." Dr. James De Gordon, Clinical Professor at Georgetown University School of Medicine

It has become increasingly evident that the food we eat has a profound effect on how our brain works. The standard American diet (SAD) is full of simple carbohydrates and simple sugars that cause many people to feel sluggish, spacey, emotional, and even depressed. Andrew Weil, MD, author of *Spontaneous Happiness*, states that modern, industrial, processed food is a possible cause for the depression epidemic and that "industrial food fails to provide our bodies with protective nutrients most abundant in vegetables and fruits."

In the following story a mother and daughter team up to improve their brain and general health.

Better Diet for a Better Brain—Georgie W.

My mom, Rose, had a stroke in her late eighties. Her brain power was greatly diminished, her thinking was fuzzy, and she lacked focus. She was also struggling with persistent depression. My mom's diet mostly consisted of sugar, starches, salt, cheese, boxed soups, and steaks.

As for me, I was tired all the time so was working with a naturopathic doctor and trying to regain my strength. I also had thyroid problems. I had been feeling fatigued and down like I didn't have all my spark plugs firing. Nothing seemed to help. My diet consisted of lots of carbs. I often perked myself up with cookies and coffee to try and stay awake.

After my mom's mini stroke, I did some research and made adjustments to our diet. I started buying all organic food and began eating more vegetables. Lots of vegetables! I made sure that I cooked something she would like so that meal times were something to look forward to. We had protein every meal—organic protein in the form of chicken, beef, or some eggs. Not too much fish because of the mercury and possible radiation. I often made homemade soups based on bone broths.

My mom snacked on nuts, yogurt, cheese, apples, and almonds. At dinner we would have some protein, a vegetable, an occasional carb (mostly potatoes or rice).

Since she changed her diet, her thinking became sharper and clearer. She got stronger and more cheerful. She also lost thirty pounds, which was an added bonus.

To change my diet, I got off gluten and wheat and I immediately started feeling better. I also ate very few carbs. Naturally–sourced thyroid supplementation also helped out. I also lost weight.

I'm committed to keeping my mom and I healthy. Eating this way really makes a big difference. My mom now refers to me as her "health angel" and tells me, "You look after my needs." Changing our diets has been an easy and nurturing way to improve health for my mom and me. ♦

Majid Fotuhi, MD, chairman of Maryland's Neurology Institute for Brain Health and Fitness states that "The best recipe is a diet that includes brain-building nutrients such as omega-3 fatty acids, antioxidants and vitamin and mineral supplements, and steers clear of foods that promote high blood pressure, high cholesterol, obesity, and diabetes."

Following are eight tips to stave off aging, live a longer life, help you keep mentally healthy, and even make you smarter.

1. **Adopt a brain healthy diet.** The food we eat has a profound effect on how our brain works. Lean protein, vegetables and fruits, nuts, olive oil and coconut oil, and foods rich in omega-3 fatty acids are essential to brain function.

Omega-3 rich foods or a high-quality omega-3 (EPA/DHA) supplement have shown significant improvements in symptoms of depression, aggression, and mental disorders as well as protection against early cognitive decline and even early Alzheimer's disease.

2. **Stay physically active.** Physical exercise is essential for maintaining good blood flow to the brain as well as to encourage new brain cells. It also can significantly reduce the risk of heart attack, stroke, and diabetes, and thereby protect against those risk factors for

Alzheimer's and other dementias. Aerobic workouts deliver oxygen to the brain and can reduce the risk of dementia and slow its progression if it starts. Exercise facilities neuroplasticity, the brain's ability to reorganize itself by forming new neural connections throughout life.

3. **Manage your body weight.** Being overweight in the prime of life can promote excess inflammation and free radical production—two enemies of a healthy brain. A long-term study of 1,500 adults found that those who were obese in middle age were twice as likely to develop dementia in later life. Adopt an overall healthy food lifestyle, rather than a short-term diet, and eat in moderation.

4. **Avoid head trauma.** Use protective headgear when engaged in physical activities such as bicycling, horseback riding, rock climbing, skiing, and skating. Wear a seat belt. Guard against falls by using handrails, watching out for tripping hazards, and taking other precautions. One head injury can ruin a life!

5. **Protect your brain.** Protecting the brain from pollution, sleep deprivation, and stress is of utmost importance for optimizing its function.

Current brain imaging research has shown that many chemicals are toxic to brain function. Alcohol, drugs of abuse, nicotine, too much caffeine, and many medications decrease blood flow to the brain. When blood flow is decreased the brain cannot work as efficiently.

6. **Exercise your mind.** Your brain is like a muscle. Use it or lose it! Every time you learn something new your brain makes a new connection and enhances blood flow and activity in the brain. If you go for long periods without learning something new you start to lose some of the connections in the brain and you begin to struggle more with memory and learning.

7. **Relax your mind.** For years, scientists have known that simple memory exercises can enhance a variety of cognitive functions. It now appears that meditation is even more effective when it comes to strengthening the neural circuits in your brain. In addition, focusing

on your breath while your belly naturally rises and falls brings a relaxation state to the brain.

8. **Thoughts matter.** The thoughts that go through your mind, moment by moment, have a significant impact on how your brain works. Research by Mark George, MD, and colleagues at the National Institutes of Health demonstrated that happy, hopeful thoughts have an overall calming effect on the brain, while negative thoughts inflame brain areas often involved with depression and anxiety. Your thoughts do matter.

A study was conducted on the activity of the brain in women under three different conditions: happy thoughts, neutral thoughts, and sad thoughts. During sad thoughts, he saw a significant increase in deep limbic system (DLS) activity. This increase in the DLS is associated with depression, dysthymia, and negativity. During the happy thoughts, the women demonstrated a cooling (lowering) of the deep limbic system.

Food Facts for the Brain

1. **Increasing water intake helps your brain.** Since your brain is about 80% water, you need adequate water to hydrate your brain. Even slight dehydration can raise stress hormones which can damage your brain over time. Drink at least half your body weight in water a day. For example if you weigh 150 pounds try to drink 75 ounces of water per day. It is best to have your liquids unpolluted with artificial sweeteners, sugar, caffeine, or alcohol. You can use herbal, non-caffeinated tea and make unsweetened iced tea. Green tea is also good for brain function as it contains chemicals that enhance mental relaxation and alertness. The amino acid L-theanine increases the activity of the neurotransmitter GABA, which has anti-anxiety effects.

2. **Eating less can increase brain size.** Mounting evidence suggests that in order to grow a bigger brain, many of us should be eating less. Several studies support this conclusion. Just a 25% reduction in calories over one month's time can have a profound effect on boosting memory.

3. **Omega-3 fatty acids** found in fish (salmon, mackerel, sardines, herring) make up a large portion of the gray matter of the brain. The fat in your brain forms cell membranes and plays a vital role in how our cells function. According to research in the last few years, diets rich in omega-3 fatty acids may help promote a healthy emotional balance and positive mood in later years, possibly because DHA is a main component of the brain's synapses.

4. **Antioxidants are essential.** A number of studies have shown that dietary intake of antioxidants from fruits and vegetables significantly reduces the risk of developing cognitive impairment. When a cell converts oxygen into energy, tiny molecules called free radicals are made. When produced in normal amounts, free radicals work to rid the body of harmful toxins, thereby keeping it healthy. When produced in toxic amounts, free radicals damage the body's cellular machinery, resulting in cell death and tissue damage. This process is called oxidative stress. Vitamin E, vitamin C, and beta carotene inhibit the production of free radicals. The best antioxidant fruits and vegetables are kale, collard greens, chard, blueberries, blackberries, cranberries, strawberries, spinach, raspberries, brussels sprouts, plums, broccoli, beets, avocados, oranges, red grapes, red bell peppers, cherries, and kiwi.

5. **Protein is brain food.** Protein in our diet enhances brain performance as it provides amino acids that make up our neurotransmitters. Think of neurotransmitters as biochemical messengers whose job it is to carry signals from one brain cell to another. These brain cells then transmit various signals to the different parts of the body to carry out their individual tasks. These messengers work to keep our minds and memory sharp.

6. **Protein is essential for our happiness.** When we don't eat enough good protein, the brain can't produce enough neurotransmitters such as serotonin, which is one of the main chemicals which regulates our moods. Eating good sources of protein such as organic meat, fish, eggs, nuts, seeds, and dairy (if well tolerated) Helps to boost our levels of serotonin and dopamine. This

boosts energy, mental clarity, and makes us feel happier as well as regulates pain, reduces anxiety, and initiates deep sleep.

7. **Choose 20-25 healthy foods for a healthy brain.** To stick with a "brain healthy" nutritional plan, it's essential to have great choices. Choosing 20-25 foods each week that are nutrient dense will help you consume powerful antioxidants, lean protein, high fiber carbohydrates, and good fat. We recommend five to nine servings of fruits and vegetables a day.

Dementia/Alzheimer's

Dementia is a loss of brain function caused by brain disease or injury and marked by memory disorders, personality changes, and impaired reasoning. Alzheimer's disease (AD) is one form of dementia that gradually gets worse over time. It affects memory, thinking, and behavior.

Here are tips for preventing dementia/Alzheimer's.

1. Avoid or eliminate any sources of aluminum exposure in cookware, utensils or foil, underarm deodorant, drinking water, and any juices and drinks packaged in aluminum–lined cartons.

2. If possible, have silver mercury dental amalgam fillings removed from your teeth in proper sequence with a biological dentist. (Mercury can leak from fillings and contribute to toxic load that can have an effect on the brain).

3. Have bodywork done such as craniosacral, applied kinesiology, chiropractic, and osteopathic care which can improve the efficiency of the flow of the nerve supply and increased oxygen and blood carrying nutrients to the brain.

4. Drinking enough water is of utmost importance. This rehydrating is very important to help compensate for the shrinkage that occurs in the brain of Alzheimer patients.

5. Eat a wide variety of foods. Rotating your foods lightens the load on your immune system.

6. Limit your consumption of alcohol, caffeine, sugar, and foods that are refined, processed or filled with chemicals, artificial colorings

and preservatives. Replace them with organically grown, pesticide free, whole foods.

Although there are many factors that could cause the following symptoms, a brain-related issue could be a possible cause.

Are you concerned about your memory? Do you feel tired and sluggish? Do you struggle with mental clarity after a meal? Are you prone to feeling depressed? If you answered yes to any of these questions, then consider these suggestions.

Start by making dietary changes and see what you notice. You may be sensitive to an excess of starchy carbs that break down like simple sugar. A balance of quality protein, good fats and vegetables will help sustain mental clarity and energy. Perhaps you would greatly benefit by increasing omega-3s in your diet.

You may be dehydrated and need to increase your water intake. Staying hydrated is very important to help compensate for the shrinkage that occurs in the brain with age. Try to get some form of exercise daily.

In Conclusion

Over the last 20 years, studies have shown that the brain has the capacity to change in response to positive or negative events. This is called Neuroplasticity. As a result, we now know that by following the tips in this chapter we can change our brains and lead happier and healthier lives.

CHAPTER 19
GUT-BRAIN CONNECTION

All disease begins in the gut.
—Hippocrates, the Father of Medicine

Have you experienced having "butterflies" in your stomach or had a "gut–wrenching" experience? There is a reason we use these expressions. A person's stomach or intestinal distress can be the cause of—or the product of—anxiety, stress, depression, or poor eating habits.

Nourishing your gut flora is extremely important, from birth through your entire life, because you have two brains, one inside your skull and one in your gut. These two organs are actually created out of the same type of tissue!

The concept that brain issues can be solved by targeting the digestive system and that gut problems can be helped by balancing the microbes in the gut is increasingly reinforced by cutting-edge science.

Anxiety can cause constipation, diarrhea, or nausea. Depression can change appetite. The connection may have been established, but scientists thought communication was one way: it traveled from the brain to the gut, and not the other way around.

But now, a new understanding of the trillions of microbes living in our guts reveals that this communication process goes two ways: gut to brain and brain to gut. By showing that changing bacteria in the gut can change behavior and how we feel, new research may transform the way we understand—and treat—a variety of brain issues.

When the fetus develops, part of the tissue turns into the central nervous system and the other develops into your enteric nervous system, which is part of the autonomic nervous system. The autonomic nervous system consists of neurons that govern the function of the gastrointestinal system. Neurons are cells that carry messages between the brain and other parts of the body which is the basis of the nervous system. The vagus nerve, a cranial nerve, runs from your brain stem down to your abdomen. It forms part of the involuntary nervous system that commands unconscious body procedures, such as keeping the heart rate constant and controlling food digestion.

The right combination of stomach microbes can be crucial for a healthy mind. And a healthy mind is crucial for a healthy gut. A troubled intestine can send signals to the brain, just as a troubled brain can send signals to the gut. Therefore, a person's stomach or intestinal distress can be the cause or the product of anxiety, stress, or depression.

Dr. Greenblatt, psychiatrist, is founder and medical director of Comprehensive Psychiatric Resources and medical director of Eating Disorder Services at Walden Behavioral Care. He states that "The gut is really your second brain, there are more neurons in the GI tract than anywhere else except the brain."

How I Made My Gut-Brain Connection—Sheri M.

When I was thirteen years old, with the usual complexities of parent and child relationships, I had some anxieties and worries that manifested in my gut as ulcerative colitis. As a result, I was advised by my doctor to cut back on some extracurricular activities and include more down time into my busy schedule of chorus, drama production, and drill team practice. I did more reading, light exercise, and just "hanging out." At that time I did not have the tools to deal with emotional issues and symptoms would come and go depending on what was going on in my life.

Over time, I began noticing the direct connection between emotions and intestinal flare–ups. If I was going through a more stressful period, I would have more intestinal issues.

Over the years, I found relaxation techniques to be particularly beneficial for stress reduction and reducing symptoms. Meditation, deep breathing, yoga, and a healthy diet have kept symptoms at bay and enabled me to successfully manage this condition. ♦

Facts

1. Your gut is home to countless bacteria, both good and bad. These bacteria outnumber the cells in your body by at least ten to one. Maintaining the ideal balance of good and bad bacteria forms the foundation for good health—physical, mental, and emotional.

2. Your gut bacteria are vulnerable to your diet and lifestyle.

3. Bacterial colonies residing in your gut may play key roles in the development of cancer, asthma, allergies, obesity, diabetes, autoimmune diseases, and even conditions like ADHD, autism, and depression.

4. Stress and negative emotions such as depression or other psychological factors can affect movement and contractions of the GI tract, cause inflammation, or make you more susceptible to infection.

5. Your gut literally serves as your second brain, and even produces more of the neurotransmitter serotonin—known to have a beneficial influence on your mood—than your brain does.

Tips for Reducing Stress and Improving Your Gut Health

1. **Avoid processed, refined foods in your diet.** If you eat sugar, refined grains, genetically engineered foods (GMO), and processed foods and beverages, your gut bacteria are going to be compromised as these foods will destroy healthy microflora and feed yeast and unfriendly bacteria (undesirable bacteria that produce toxins in the body).

2. **Take a high-quality probiotic supplement.** Taking a high-quality probiotic supplement is recommended. Researchers state that probiotics may profoundly affect the brain-gut interactions and reduce the development of stress-induced disorders in both the upper and lower gastrointestinal tract. If you must take antibiotics (which interfere with the ratio of good bacteria versus bad bacteria in your

colon), we recommend that you temporarily increase your dosage of probiotics to correct this problem.

3. **Eat fermented foods** such as kefir, plain yogurt, and fermented vegetables such as sauerkraut and kimchi.

4. **Physical exercise** is very helpful for stress relief and clearing your mind.

5. **Relaxation exercises** such as prayer, yoga, meditation, deep breathing, and positive visualization can work to turn off the stress response, in which gut changes come about in response to thoughts and feelings. (Read final chapter for more on relaxation.)

In Conclusion

We have two brains, one in the gut and one in the brain. Studies reveal that communication goes back and forth between the two. Since the stomach microbes affect the mind, it's important to maintain a balance of bacteria, through proper diet, taking probiotics, getting exercise, and relaxing the mind through meditation or other stress reduction techniques.

CHAPTER 20
CANCER–PART 1

I believe in hope. I believe in believing.
Believing that there is light through all this darkness.
—Lynne Knowlton

The number of people being diagnosed with cancer is on the rise. In the distant past, it was rare to have a friend or relative with this disease. These days, it's quite common to have several friends or relatives who have dealt with or died from cancer. Nearly half of all men and one-third of women will at some point in their lives develop cancer, according to American Cancer Society estimates. Here's a glimpse into the history of cancer:

- In the early 1900s, one in 20 people developed cancer.
- In the 1940s, one in 16 people developed cancer.
- In the 1970s, one in 10 people developed cancer.
- Today, one in three people develop cancer.

According to the Center for Disease Control (CDC), about 1.66 million new cancer cases were diagnosed in 2013.

What Is Cancer?

Cancer begins as a single abnormal cell that begins to multiply out of control. Groups of such cells form tumors and invade healthy tissue, often spreading to other parts of the body.

Carcinogens are substances that promote the development of cancerous cells. They come from certain foods, the air, and even from within the body. Most carcinogens are neutralized before damage can occur, but sometimes they attack the cell's genetic material (DNA) and alter it. It can take years for a noticeable tumor to develop. During this time, compounds known as inhibitors can keep the cells from growing.

Cancer Research and Prevention

Cancer is big business. Of its multi-million-dollar resources, the cancer industry is spending very little on prevention strategies, such as diet, exercise, and obesity education. Profits are spent instead on treating cancer (chemotherapy, radiation, diagnostics, and surgeries). Each year the United States spends billions of dollars on how to treat cancer. We have some of the best cancer specialists and cancer treatment centers in the world. Yet, the United States falls short when it comes to cancer prevention. Cancer research funding in the U.S. spends too much money on treatment and too little spent on prevention. Traditional methods for treating cancer (radiation and chemotherapy) do not always prolong life. The best approach to cancer is prevention.

Is Cancer Preventable?

According to the Berkeley Wellness Report, 65% of all cancers might not have occurred if Americans had never smoked, had healthier diets, and exercised more. Only 10% are caused by inherited genes that increase cancer risk. The Harvard Report on Cancer Prevention lists diet and smoking as the highest contributors to cancer. Other factors that contribute to cancer are stress and the thousands of chemicals we are exposed to throughout our lives, beginning in utero.

The Importance of Fruits and Vegetables

Fruits and vegetables contain antioxidants and cancer-fighting substances. They are high in fiber as well. Antioxidants are naturally-occurring molecules believed to fight against the action of free radicals, which adversely alter lipids, proteins, and DNA, and trigger disease.

Carotenoids, the pigment that gives fruits and vegetables their dark colors, have been shown to help prevent cancer. Beta-carotene, present in dark green and yellow vegetables, helps protect against lung cancer and may help prevent cancers of the bladder, mouth, larynx, esophagus, breast, and other parts of the body.

Vitamin C, found in citrus fruits and many vegetables, may lower risks for cancers of the esophagus and stomach. It acts as an antioxidant, neutralizing cancer-causing chemicals that form in the body. It also blocks the conversion of nitrates to cancer-causing nitrosamines in the stomach.

Plants also contain phytochemicals—substances that may help your body fight cancer. The five major classes of compounds that occur in fruits and vegetables as natural blocking agents against carcinogens are phenols, indoles, flavones, cumines, and isothiocyanates. These neutralizing agents prevent carcinogens from reaching critical target sites within the cell. The vegetables specifically helpful for reducing the risk of cancer are the cruciferous vegetables: broccoli, cabbage, brussels sprouts, mustard greens, kale, and cauliflower.

Dr. Dean Ornish, clinical professor of medicine at the University of California, San Francisco, showed that after just three months on an intensive lifestyle program, including a whole-foods, plant-based diet, over 500 genes that regulate cancer were beneficially affected, either turning off the cancer-causing genes or turning on the cancer-protective genes. There is no existing medication that can do that.

As an oncology dietician, Tinrin Chew advises cancer patients about the "tremendous power of food" and how it impacts their genetic expression—both positively and negatively. For twenty years she worked at Alta Bates Hospital where she watched people with cancer survive or die, stating that "food has tremendous impact on your well–being and survivorship." She emphasizes eating a wide variety of fruits and vegetables, a "rainbow" of colors, and to "rotate, rotate, rotate" to ensure having a well-rounded diet.

One of Chew's patients, Sheila, graciously shares her inspiring cancer story and the measures she took to not only survive cancer but to thrive.

My Cancer Story—Sheila H.

On July 7, 2007, I was diagnosed with stage III breast cancer and type 2 diabetes. It was a dark day indeed. Fear gripped me and held on with a vengeance. I had a sense, though, that I needed more than a team of specialized doctors, but I wasn't sure exactly what form that support would take. The day I signed the papers for the chemo, I felt as if I had signed my death warrant. At my oncologist's office, I asked the doctor for help, not to kill the cancer, but for emotional support for the woman inside of me who was suffering in the throes of the biggest challenge of her life. I was given some pamphlets to read.

A week later I saw an endocrinologist in order to better understand diabetes. He advised me to deal with the cancer first and that he would support and educate me through the diabetes. He did just that.

The evening I told my children about my diagnosis, I made a promise to them that I would fight to survive. That was my first motivational step.

Secondly, it wasn't a "what" but a "who" who motivated me to make some drastic and life changing adjustments for my health and, ultimately, for the rest of my life. That person, recommended to me by my endocrinologist, was a nutritionist specializing in oncology named Tinrin Chew, registered dietician. She took the time to educate me about my cancer and how to survive the treatment. It would necessitate my understanding the purpose of chemotherapy drugs, how they worked, and what I could do to survive their toxic side effects. It was this education that reintroduced some semblance of control into my daily life. Tinrin spent hours helping me design a daily diet to protect and boost my immune system, control my diabetes, and give me hope for survival.

Below are the dietary changes I made based on her recommendations. First, I worked to decrease or eliminate non-organic meat and dairy products, grilling and barbequing, alcohol, salt, inactivity, and exposure to hazardous materials (especially in makeup).

I completely eliminated all white flour in bread, pasta, and baked goods, as well as white rice and all sugars, white or brown (except natural sugar in fruit).

I increased consumption of organic vegetables and fruit (monitored due to diabetes, no fruit juices), vitamins C and D3, fiber, nuts—especially walnuts—and seeds, flax, and whole grains such as brown rice, buckwheat, quinoa, whole oats, and millet. This diet addressed both my cancer and diabetes.

I shopped locally for fresh vegetables, especially dark and leafy greens along with small amounts of vegetable juices. Over time, I worked up to exercising one to two hours a day: walking outside or on my treadmill, riding my bike, and lifting weights. I am a three-year student of QiGong (a practice of aligning body, breath, and mind for health and meditation). I drank 64 ounces of purified water daily in addition to lots of green tea.

My new diet:

- I ate two to three servings/day of cruciferous vegetables: broccoli, cauliflower, cabbage, brussels sprouts, kale, mustard greens, collards, turnips, bok choy, and arugula. I also ate carrots and mushrooms.
- I ate one to two servings/day of onions, garlic, leeks, shallots, green onions, and pearl onions. I also ate two to three servings of sea vegetables or twelve kelp tablets especially when receiving radiation. I ate nori and kombu seaweeds and drank gallons of miso soup. (Miso is a fermented soybean paste with beneficial microorganisms and provides protection from radiation and lowers the risks of breast cancer.) I increased fish because it's a good source of protein and omega-3.

I posted the new eating regime on my refrigerator. I was also adjusting to testing my blood sugars; it was a daunting task. I felt ill, weak, and shook so much that I could not make the meter work. My husband went with me to meetings with Tinrin, who suggested I make a daily plan for meals and exercise. Another team of women friends asked what they could cook for me, which led me to Rebecca Katz's books, *One Bite at a Time* and *The Cancer Fighting Kitchen*. The primary tool introduced in these books is flavor, which is vital when taste buds are severely impaired by chemotherapy. I attended Rebecca's cooking workshops where I learned by cooking and tasting that, in Rebecca's words, "Great taste and great nutrition can joyfully coexist on the dinner table."

Fresh vegetables from the farmers' market (devoid of pesticides) became my most sought-after foods. Gradually, I lusted for veggies I had never tried. My friends made me gallons of "Magic Broth" soup found in *One Bite at a Time*. I literally lived on this vegetable-based broth all through chemotherapy.

After a chemotherapy infusion, I had a three-hour window before I began to feel poorly. I would troll the grocery aisles reading labels and vowing to never purchase another processed food item again. I also rewarded myself by buying a new stylish head wrap for my balding head!

Now I was on a roll making other changes all under the umbrella of caring for myself. I began walking for exercise. My meditation teacher, a most dear 82-year old Holocaust survivor, called me every day to ask if I had moved from the couch to at least walk around my backyard. I was encouraged to breathe, lift a leaf, find a ladybug, and express gratitude for the moment of that discovery.

After surgery, radiation, and months of recovery, I enrolled in a QiGong class and found a community of cancer survivors who were so uplifting that no matter how badly I felt, I dragged myself to attend.

Gratitude seeped into the cavities where cancer had been, and for the first time, I found myself truly believing that I could survive with dignity, hope, and appreciation. I wanted to share this newfound goodness so I began volunteering as a patient navigator at my cancer center. It was a humbling experience.

A writing teacher I knew encouraged me to journal about my year of recovery, and for the first time, I started writing poetry at night when sleep eluded me. Thus, I was granted permission to cry and spit out anger, sadness, and fear. Ever so slowly the burden of having cancer and going through the rigorous treatment lifted, and I recognized the gift of transformation.

Feeling different came after looking different. I had had a mastectomy and my hair was gone, but I had also lost seventy-five pounds. Amazingly, I liked how I looked because I had achieved a dramatic weight loss. All through the rigors of chemotherapy, surgery, and radiation, I struggled to eat anything (what a surprise that was!), but I found that when my appetite gradually returned I naturally sought out foods with a high nutritional load. Having diabetes required that I reduce carbs, increase fiber, and eat tons of vegetables at all meals, which helped control my blood sugar. Regular exercise contributed to weight loss and maintenance.

I emerged from a year of cancer treatment with more energy than I'd had in years. I had entered a new phase in my life. I was alive, cancer-free, and healthier. More importantly, I knew how to remain so.

Being a cancer survivor was challenging, though, with endless doctor appointments, shopping, and cooking more thoughtfully, and learning to advocate for myself in social situations. The demands of change descended upon me, and I was faced with the challenge of depression that many post-cancer patients face. But I realized that I had the tools to fight this, too. And so I ramped up by moving from walking to long-distance hiking.

My son challenged me to climb a mountain with him. And so, in 2012, I bought hiking poles, trained for six months, and in August I flew to Colorado where my son and I hiked thirty miles and ascended a 14,000-foot mountain. Standing on the mountain was a life-altering event just like the cancer, but this time I cried with gratitude, hope, and a desire to live in the moment every day.

When I returned to California, I realized that I had indeed carved out a new way of living. I re-evaluated all aspects of my life. When a new administrator at the school where I taught created a toxic work environment, I set limits and chose self-care first...so I resigned. It was scary but ultimately led me to a new job teaching sign language to seniors—a most enriching and rewarding experience. Life is good!◆

By using the expertise of a nutritionist, accepting support from friends, meditating and practicing QiGong, journaling to help express her feelings, and getting involved with a community of survivors, she slowly lifted her burden of cancer. Today, seven years after her diagnosis, Sheila remains cancer free.

Dietary Changes That Will Lower Your Cancer Risk

You don't all of a sudden "get cancer." The chances are that you, and even your children, have a few cancer cells lurking in your body. This is why we emphasize beginning the anticancer diet, in early life, since some cancer cells develop very slowly over decades.

The consumption of some foods actually contributes to the development of cancer while other foods lessen the risk. For example, omega-6 fatty acids accelerate the growth of human prostate tumors.

The researchers pointed out that the rate of prostate cancer in the United States has increased steadily along with intake of omega-6, suggesting a possible link between diet and prostate cancer. Specific cancer prevention guidelines are outlined later in this chapter.

The following story shows how changing one's diet can reverse pre-cancer.

How Simple Dietary Changes Squelched Cancer Cells
—Rosa Z.

My husband has always been active and healthy. He enjoys tennis, golf, and playing with our young granddaughter. Three years ago, he was diagnosed with carcinogenic cells on his prostate.

When confronted with the idea that he may have prostate cancer, he started eating healthier. He eliminated all sugars, white flour, red meat, white pasta, white rice, and coffee from his diet. He was very serious and disciplined about his new healthy way of eating.

He started eating sugar-free cereals for breakfast, organic soup for lunch, and lots of broccoli, hummus, salmon, and organic chicken with vegetables. Instead of soda, he drank low-sodium mineral water with pomegranate juice.

He was scheduled for another biopsy in two months. In the meantime, he continued eating healthy.

When he went for his second biopsy, he told the doctor about his new healthy eating habits. The doctor smiled and said, "Of course, we all hope for the best." We, but we could tell he was not convinced that this new change in diet would make a difference.

We waited three weeks before the doctor called my husband with the results. To our surprise, the results came out negative for carcinogenic cells. My husband's new diet reversed those potentially cancerous cells. We were both very happy!

It's been five years since that day. My husband continues to enjoy the benefits of eating this healthy, new way. His annual checkups have been normal and healthy, too. We are grateful for our new way of life!◆

Top 12 Cancer Prevention Guidelines

1. **Organic vegetables and fruit.** Increase your intake with a variety of fresh and preferably locally grown. Five to seven –servings a day is recommended.

2. **Protein and fat.** Eat high quality proteins and fats such as those received from organic eggs from pastured hens, high-quality

(organic whenever possible) meat, salmon, nuts, seeds, avocados, and coconut oil.

3. **Supplements.** Scientific evidence shows you can decrease your cancer risk by supplementing with vitamin D, vitamin C, curcumin (turmeric), and resveratrol.

4. **Plant-based omega-3.** Consume sources such as ground flaxseeds, chia seeds, hemp seeds, walnuts, dark green leafy vegetables, and krill oil.

5. **Regular exercise.** Thirty minutes a day increases survivorship by 50%. Exercise lowers your risk for cancer by reducing elevated insulin levels which are associated with an increased risk of cancer.

6. **Good sleep.** Good sleep is required for optimal health and directly impacts your immune function. Get at least –seven to eight hours. Impaired immune function can raise your cancer risk.

7. **Reduce exposure to environmental toxins** in personal care products, pesticides, household chemical cleaners, synthetic air fresheners, and air pollution.

8. **Use devices to protect yourself from electromagnetic radiation** produced by computers, cell phones, cell phone towers, and WiFi. (Learn more in the Electromagnetic Radiation chapter).

9. **Stress Management.** Stress from all causes is a major contributor to disease. Practice stress reduction techniques such as yoga, tai chi, walking, and meditation.

10. **Increase your fiber intake.** Good sources are beans and legumes, fruits and vegetables, oat bran, prunes, flaxseed, and whole grains.

11. **Think positive thoughts**. The Mayo Clinic states that positive thinking and optimism are key components to good health and effective stress management.

12. **Practice forgiveness.** According to the Harvard Women's Health Watch, forgiving those who hurt you can improve your mental and physical well-being.

Avoid the Following for Cancer Prevention

1. **Trans fatty acids.** Stay away from imitation fats in shortenings, margarines, and most commercial baked goods and snack foods. These are strongly associated with cancer of the lungs and reproductive organs.

2. **Rancid fats.** Industrial processing creates rancidity (free radicals) in commercial vegetable oils (processed seed oils like soybean oil, sunflower oil, corn oil, canola oil, cottonseed oil, and safflower oil). Just because they are "vegetable" oils, doesn't mean they're good for you.

3. **Omega-6 fatty acids.** Although needed in small amounts, an excess can contribute to cancer. Dangerously high levels of omega-6 fatty acids are due to the overuse of vegetable oils such as soybean, corn, and sunflower that are found in many processed foods in modern diets.

4. **MSG.** This chemical has been associated with brain cancer. Found in almost all processed foods, even when "MSG" does not appear on the label. Flavorings, spice mixes, and hydrolyzed protein contain MSG.

5. **Aspartame.** This artificial sweetener in diet foods and beverages has been associated with brain cancer.

6. **GMOs.** Avoid genetically modified foods as they can be carcinogenic.

7. **Pesticides.** Pesticide exposure has been linked to a number of chronic diseases including cancer.

8. **Hormones.** Some scientists believe that human consumption of estrogen from hormone-fed beef can result in cancer. Additionally, phytoestrogens in soy disrupt endocrine function and have the potential to promote breast cancer in adult women.

9. **Artificial flavorings and food coloring.** These have been associated with various types of cancers, especially when consumed in large amounts in a diet of junk food. Though approved by the FDA, red food dye, referred to as Red 40 and Allura Red, may contribute to cancer in humans and could trigger hyperactivity in children, according to the Center for Science in the Public Interest (CSPI).

10. **Refined carbohydrates.** Sugar, high fructose corn syrup, and white flour are devoid of nutrients. The body uses up nutrients from other foods to process refined carbohydrates. Tumor growth is associated with sugar consumption.

11. **Frying or grilling.** Frying or grilling your meat and fish at high heat can form carcinogenic chemicals. Cooking at low temperatures is safer.

12. **Anger, resentment, and unforgiveness.** Studies show that negative emotions weaken your body, while positive emotions strengthen your body. (See final chapter for ways to release and let go of negative emotions).

Fat Consumption and Cancer

Controversy exists concerning the relationship between fat consumption and cancer. Some fats, like those rich in omega-3s, actually help prevent cancer and inflammation. Fat from hydrogenated fats (trans fats) contributes to cancer.

The well-known Dr. Barry Sears, who battled and survived colon cancer, was mainly concerned about how to prevent getting cancer again. As part of his treatment program, he consulted top cancer specialists and visited one of the top cancer centers in the world. When asked what he could do nutritionally to lower his chances of having a "return visit," the oncologist glibly said, "Don't eat too many hamburgers." Such was the extent of nutritional counseling for cancer prevention. That's when he realized that a cancer survivor is more motivated than even the top cancer specialists to do his homework on preventing cancer.

Dr. Sears' philosophy points to inflammation as the underlying cause of chronic disease, and how our diet can either reduce inflammation or increase it. He promotes the Zone Diet, rich in long-chain omega-3 fatty acids which he considers "an ideal life-long eating strategy to lower the risk of cancer." (More about omega fatty acids in Chapter 24 "Good Fats, Bad Fats.")

Part of the controversy concerning fat and cancer is whether animal products contribute to cancer cells in the body. The China Study by T. Colin Campbell, PhD, concluded that "People who ate the most animal-based foods got the most chronic disease. People who ate the most plant-based foods were the healthiest."

There is controversy surrounding the conclusions of The China Study. Those who researched The China Study got a very different picture and feel it has fundamental flaws.

In his studies, Campbell showed that casein (the main protein in dairy) promotes cancer in rats. In fact, he was able to turn the cancer gene on and off simply by feeding them casein. Then, he concluded that all animal proteins have this same effect. He made the assumption that because dairy protein turned on the cancer gene, that meat protein does the same thing. This is the major controversy regarding the China Study—whether animal protein in the form of meat is also associated with cancer.

Many studies link eating meat with various types of cancer. Other studies link consuming dairy with various types of cancer. So what does one eat to avoid cancer? The real factors to consider are: do health conscious grass-fed meat eaters also consume organic fruits and vegetables, exercise and avoid processed meat? Diet and lifestyle choices are equally important.

Just as a vegetarian diet is not always right for everyone, frequently eating large portions of meat is not healthy either. When deciding whether or not meat is right for you, consider these questions:

1. Is the meat organic or "conventional"? Conventional meats can be loaded with pesticides, hormones, antibiotics, and other chemicals.

2. What's the animal eating? Green grass or genetically modified grains?

3. How's the animal being treated? Humanely or abusively? Overcrowded conditions to produce the highest output at the lowest cost? This requires the use of antibiotics and pesticides to mitigate the spread of disease exacerbated by the crowded living conditions. Cows

free to roam the land, eating grass and treated humanely, will produce the healthier product.

4. Is the meat processed? Processed meat can contain nitrates, preservatives, or additives. Eating processed meats has been highly associated with an increased risk of colon cancer.

5. Is the meat cooked at high temperatures? Whether grilling, frying, or broiling, high temps create unhealthy chemicals that can be carcinogenic. Grilling under high heat (such as searing or flame-cooking meat to well done) can release carcinogens into the meat called heterocyclic amines, which can damage cellular DNA. Poach, bake, stew, boil, steam, sauté, or slowly cook your foods over low heat instead. The good news is that these chemicals are not released when grilling fruits or vegetables.

What about Dairy?

The saturated fat in meat is different than the saturated fat in dairy. In the Kaiser study referred to below, the issue of estrogen in dairy is addressed.

According to a 2013 study conducted by scientists at Kaiser Permanente, published in the *Journal of the National Cancer Institute*, breast cancer survivors consuming cow dairy with a high fat content have a higher risk of dying from breast cancer than women eating little to no high-fat dairy.

The researchers followed 1,893 women diagnosed with early-stage invasive breast cancer for nearly twelve years. At the end of the study, the women who had consumed the most high-fat dairy foods (more than one serving per day) were found to have a 49% higher risk of dying from breast cancer than those who consumed the least high-fat dairy (less than half a serving per day).

According to this study, the theory is that it's not the fat in the dairy, it's what's *in* the fat. It's the hormone estrogen that links dairy fat to breast cancer. Much of the cow milk we drink today is from pregnant cows, whose estrogen and progesterone levels are markedly elevated. By consuming milk from these cows, humans can increase their own estrogen levels, creating an environment that is conducive to breast cancer but that has also been linked to prostate, endometrial, and ovarian cancers. A report from Harvard suggests that milk from factory farms may be associated with hormone-related cancers because of the industrial agricultural practice of milking a cow throughout her pregnancy. The later in pregnancy a cow is, the more hormones appear in her milk. Milk from a cow in the late stage of pregnancy contains up to thirty-three times as much of a signature estrogen compound (estrone sulfate) as milk from a cow following pregnancy, as well as much higher levels of other hormones.

When it comes to dairy, we recommend that enjoying small amounts of dairy is better because of the two main issues: estrogen and casein. Eat organic whenever possible and choose varieties such as sheep (feta cheese), goat cheese, or kefir (fermented milk containing beneficial bacteria). Some studies say this will reduce the risk of breast cancer and bladder cancer. More research is needed.

Excess Body Weight: Higher Cancer Risk

Excess body fat is a risk factor for cancer, especially colorectal cancer.

Obesity is also a risk factor for breast cancer because increased fat tissue raises circulating estrogen. Women who maintain normal weight, consume a high-fiber diet and steer clear of a high sugar, refined carb diet tend to have lower blood levels of estrogen and therefore are less prone to breast cancer. Men who are obese have a higher rate of prostate cancer.

Higher Fiber: Lower Incidence of Cancer

In all the research between food and cancer, the evidence for a relationship between a high fiber diet and lower chances of colorectal cancer is the most conclusive. It follows common sense as well. Fiber moves potential carcinogens through the intestines faster, decreasing the contact time between carcinogens and the intestinal wall. The less exposure to carcinogens, the less chance of colon cancer.

Fiber promotes the growth of healthy bacteria in the intestines, which crowd out the undesirable bacteria. Besides lowering the risk of colorectal cancer, a high-fiber diet can lower the risk of breast cancer by binding estrogen in the bowels, thereby lessening the estrogen effect in the cells of breast tissue. Also, stomach cancer is less common on high-fiber diets.

The best anti-cancer fiber sources are: oat bran, kidney beans, garbanzo beans, navy beans, whole grains, and prunes. Get used to looking at nutrition labels to find the fiber content of foods. Simple additions to your diet can increase the amount of fiber you eat.

What about Soy Products?

Soy products are controversial. Some research suggests that soy inhibits the growth of new blood vessels necessary for tumor survival and can also protect against colon cancer. Isoflavones are said to regulate the production of sex hormones, which could help reduce the risk of prostate and breast cancer. Some studies have shown that women who eat more soy foods have less risk of breast cancer. However, other studies report on the estrogenic effects of soy, which can increase estrogen in the body and contribute to certain types of tumors. Soy beans are said to have the highest phytates levels of any grain or legume. Phytates block mineral absorption, specifically calcium, magnesium, copper, iron, and zinc. The phytates in soy are particularly resistant to cooking. Only fermentation reduces the phytates level. Research suggests that fermented soy products such as miso, kimchee, and tempeh are the healthier choices.

8 Cancer Facts

1. Diet plays a much larger role in cancer development than genes.

2. It is estimated that 70-90% of cancers are due to unhealthy diet, lifestyle and environmental factors.

3. A plant-based diet (eating a wide variety of organic, fresh fruits and vegetables, beans and legumes, and nuts and seeds daily) lowers the rate of breast, prostate, and colon cancers.

4. Omega-3 slows down tumor growth rate, decreases cell mutation and blood clots, and decreases inflammation.

5. Fiber is protective against certain forms of cancer and promotes the growth of healthy bacteria in the intestines, which crowd out the undesirable bacteria. Foods that are closest to their natural state, unrefined and unpeeled, are highest in fiber.

6. A dramatic increase in the uptake of sugar by a cell could be a cause for its becoming cancerous. Cancer cells have 400 times the ability to transport sugar into themselves.

7. Patients who receive the proper balance of healthy foods, vitamins, minerals, and nutritional supplements show a striking increase in the effectiveness of their chemotherapy and radiation treatments.

8. The World Health Organization (WHO) declares, "Radiation from cell phones can possibly cause cancer." Learn more about this in the chapter on Electromagnetic Radiation.

In Conclusion

Controversy still exists whether animal fat causes cancer. Some studies suggest it does, other research suggests it doesn't. We believe small portions of quality meat, farmed humanely, organic and grass-fed, is beneficial to your health, together with a wide variety of organic fresh fruits and vegetables.

With regard to dairy, because of casein and estrogen, hormones and antibiotics, it's best to avoid dairy for cancer prevention.

CHAPTER 21
CANCER–PART 2

A faithful friend is the medicine of life.

Being diagnosed with cancer is like no other experience. It immediately rattles our thoughts and disrupts our dreams. Our hearts and minds fill with fear. This is a normal reaction. Part of the fear comes from a lack of understanding regarding the nature of cancer.

Society's current focus with cancer is epidemiology, which infers something has been cast upon us from the outside. Another way to approach the diagnosis is to look at the endemiology of cancer, those influences coming from within the individual which may be eating.

equally significant and potentially under our control. Dr. Paul J. Rosch, president of The American Institute of Stress states, "Many times it is much more important to know what kind of patient has the disease, than what kind of disease the patient has."

The threat of cancer is so serious that every avenue needs to be explored with an open mind and not left only to the pharmaceutical and Western medical arenas.

For decades, mainstream medicine has denied the link between stress and cancer. But science is now telling us otherwise. Over the past several decades, clinical and animal research studies have confirmed that the influence of stressful emotions can lead to disease and particularly malignant growth. If we acknowledge that the mind and the body are undeniably linked, then changes in our attitudes and outlook on life also affect our physical state of well–being.

According to Dr. Leonard Coldwell, a leading cancer specialist and authority on stress-related illness, theorizes that the root cause of cancer needs to be addressed: the bad marriage, the stressful job, the continuous compromising against yourself, the lack of hope, the lack of love, the lack of self–love. While there can be outside influences that cause cancer, emotions play a key role.

Identifying stressful areas in your life is the first step toward reclaiming your health. Removing stress allows the body to do what it was designed to do: be healthy and disease free.

These coping skills can play an important role in cancer prevention and the healing process.

- a feeling of hope and optimism
- a firm belief in faith—that which brings contentment or inner peace
- a feeling of social support from family and friends
- emotional support from a therapist or support group to get in touch with suppressed emotions

Long-term studies show that these coping skills are highly effective in reducing malignancy.

Reports of cancer cures from shrines, faith healers, acupuncture, macrobiotic diets, vitamin therapy, homeopathy, and other alternative treatments abound. How can one explain the numerous well-documented cases of spontaneous remission of cancer?

In researching alternatives for healing cancer, we read her book and would like to introduce to you, Kelly Turner, PhD, researcher and psychotherapist who graduated from Harvard and UC Berkeley and specializes in integrative oncology. Dr. Turner wrote the book *Radical Remission* on her findings of one thousand cases of cancer survivors who have defied a serious or even terminal cancer diagnosis with a complete reversal of the disease.

Dr. Turner's findings suggest that there are several factors present when a person with cancer has a spontaneous remission. Here are the nine key factors that she found among nearly every radical remission survivor she studied. Only two factors had to do with the physical body and those included: (1) diet and (2) herbs and supplements.

The radical change in diet was "no sweets, no meat, no dairy, no refined foods."

The other seven factors point to emotions:

1. releasing suppressed negative emotion,
2. replacing with positive emotions,
3. tuning into your intuition,
4. connecting with your sense of spirituality,
5. feeling empowered to deal with the cancer versus feeling like a victim,
6. having a strong motive to live, and
7. getting emotional support from family and friends.

Support from Friends Made All the Difference—Pat B.

In December of 2004, I had the devastating diagnosis of breast cancer. I had a right breast mastectomy, which included removal of all lymph nodes from my underarm area.

After my surgery, I was scheduled for eight weeks of chemotherapy. Knowing that I would need help, my best friend, Sheri Miller, asked me for the phone numbers and email addresses of my many wonderful friends. She then scheduled a different friend to take me to my treatments and drive me home each day. Once we were home, the friends would visit with me for a while and often fix me something to eat. Since several friends took turns helping me, any inconvenience to them was minimal.

I can never thank Sheri and my friends enough for their kindness and for their incredible plan to help me. It truly made a difference in my ability to cope with my situation and recover from cancer.

I am now a ten-year cancer survivor and help other cancer patients on a personal level by sharing my experience. I also promote Drivers for Survivors, an organization that provides drivers for cancer patients in the Fremont Tri-City area of Northern California.

I'm sharing my story to let people know how they can help others who have cancer. For me, support from my friends and my community was crucial for my well–being, healing, and recovery. ♦

Another Way to Connect Family and Friends

Caring Bridge is a charitable 501c nonprofit organization established in 1997, which offers free personalized websites to people facing serious medical conditions, hospitalization, undergoing medical treatment, and/or recovering from a significant accident, illness, injury, or procedure.

Visitors are provided with the personal website address and password, if required, and can read updates on the patient's condition and post messages to the family.

Alternative Cancer Resources

For over thirty-five years, biochemist Stanislaw Burzynski, PhD, has been treating and curing cancer at his world-renowned cancer treatment clinic in Houston, Texas. His work is based on the natural biochemical defense system of the body, with minimal impact on healthy cells.

Dr. Burzynski won the largest legal battle against the Food & Drug Administration in American history based on his gene-targeted approach using non-toxic peptides and amino acids he discovered in the 1970s called antineoplastons. Antineoplastons are chemical compounds found normally in blood and urine. These compounds are responsible for curing some of the most incurable forms of terminal cancer.

When antineoplastons are approved, it will mark the first time in history a single scientist, not a pharmaceutical company, will hold the exclusive patent and distribution rights on a major medical breakthrough.

Burzynski, the Movie is an internationally award-winning documentary originally released in 2010 (with an extended edition released in 2011). This documentary takes the audience through a fourteen-year journey both Dr. Burzynski and his patients had to endure in order to obtain FDA-approved clinical trials for antineoplastons.

In the film, various cancer survivors tell their stories about choosing his medicines instead of surgery, chemotherapy, or radiation—with full disclosure of medical records to support their diagnosis and recovery. The information is published within the peer-reviewed medical literature.

One form of cancer, childhood brainstem glioma, has never before been cured in any scientifically controlled clinical trial in the history of medicine. Antineoplastons hold the first cures in history—dozens of them.

Burzynski's ability to successfully treat incurable cancer with such consistency has baffled the industry. Ironically, this fact had prompted numerous investigations by the Texas Medical Board, who relentlessly took Dr. Burzynski as high as the state supreme court in their failed attempt to halt his practices.

Likewise, the Food and Drug Administration engaged in four federal grand juries spanning over a decade attempting to indict Dr. Burzynski, all of which ended in no finding of fault on his behalf. For these reasons, we encourage you to check out the Burzynski Movie: Cancer Is Serious Business, to see for yourself the profound work he's doing in the field of cancer.

The National Cancer Institute's annual budget is $5.389 billion, a $174.6 million increase over 2016. According to Joseph Mercola, MD, "Much of this money goes toward the highly toxic drugs and expensive machines...the same old paradigm centered around profit."

All of Dr. Burzynski's research into antineoplastons over the past thirty-five years has been self-funded.

The Gerson Therapy

Dr. Max Gerson developed the Gerson Therapy in the 1920s. The Gerson Therapy focuses on the concept that you have the power to heal yourself, and it uses non-toxic methods, including organic foods, juicing, detoxification, and supplements, to activate the body's healing potential. Many of the success stories include people whose conventional doctors gave no hope for recovery, who were able to overcome their disease against all odds using not toxic cancer drugs but natural fruits and vegetables.

As stated by the non-profit Gerson Institute: "The Gerson Therapy is a powerful, natural treatment that boosts your body's own immune system to heal cancer, arthritis, heart disease, allergies, and many other degenerative diseases. One aspect of the Gerson Therapy that sets it apart from most other treatment methods is its all-encompassing nature.

An abundance of nutrients from thirteen fresh, organic juices are consumed every day, providing the patient with a super dose of enzymes, minerals, and nutrients. These substances then break down diseased tissue in the body, while enemas aid in eliminating the lifelong buildup of toxins from the liver. With its whole-body approach to healing, the Gerson Therapy naturally reactivates your body's magnificent ability to heal itself—with no damaging side-effects."

This system is not a miracle cure for everyone, and even the Gerson Institute states that "No treatment works for everyone, every time." But most conventional physicians offer only one route for cancer treatment—drugs, radiation and surgery—while ignoring or discounting alternative options.

Homeopathy as a Viable Alternative

In India, homeopathy is accepted as a genuine medical therapy. Homeopathy is based on the idea that "like cures like." That is, if a substance causes a symptom in a healthy person, giving the person a very small amount of the same substance may cure the illness. In theory, a homeopathic dose enhances the body's normal healing and self-regulatory processes.

Every day miracles are carried out at several homeopathic clinics in Calcutta and it was there that American researchers went to see the work for themselves.

Dr. Moshe Frankel, who was working for the MD Anderson Cancer Center in Houston, Texas, was astounded by what he witnessed. "I saw things there that I couldn't explain. Tumors shrank with nothing else other than homeopathic remedies." Two of the remedies, Carcinosin and Phytolacca, achieved as much as 80% response, indicating that they had caused apoptosis (programmed cell death) and interfered with the cancer cells' normal growth cycle. Yet, the researchers found that the surrounding healthy cells were untouched. The homeopathic remedies targeted only the cancer cells, whereas chemotherapy drugs attack all growing cells, including healthy cells.

In another study involving the homeopathic remedy Ruta 6, 127 American patients with brain tumors, half of whom were stage IV (the end-stage before death), were given Ruta with no conventional treatment. Overall, 79% of the brain-tumor patients surveyed enjoyed some benefit from Ruta.

It's perplexing why good medical studies and breakthroughs are not widely recognized or discussed in the West.

New Paradigm of Healing

The new healing paradigm is about giving patients back their power and autonomy. When you're faced with a serious health challenge, know with absolute certainty that not only is your body capable of healing but that it was designed to heal.

If we acknowledge that the mind and the body are undeniably linked, then changes in our attitudes and outlook on life affect our physical state of well-being.

Cancer is so serious a threat that every avenue needs to be explored with an open mind. Many conventional physicians offer only one route for cancer treatment—drugs, radiation, and surgery—while ignoring or discounting alternative options.

In Conclusion

Over the last hundred years, a number of natural, successful cancer treatments have been developed to treat patients in the U.S. and other countries. Homeopathy, Dr. Burzynski's antineoplastons, and the Gerson Therapy are just a few examples of innovative approaches that have been met with great success.

Viable alternative treatments are often met with opposition by the pharmaceutical and medical industries. In time, alternative methods will become more mainstream and patients will have more options when faced with treatments for cancer.

CHAPTER 22
CANCER RECOVERY STORIES

She stood in the storm and when the wind did not blow her way,
she adjusted her sails.
—Elizabeth Edwards

Below are stories from two brave women who each healed cancer in her own unique way. Both of these women are living very full, passionate lives today. May these stories serve as an inspiration to you or a loved one who is struggling with cancer.

Finding the Antidote in the Venom—Erika L.

The sun sparkled off the bay as I headed over the bridge for a recording session in Sausalito. My partner, Lisa, and I had just returned from tour and I was happy to be home. As a musician, I was used to being away for long stretches of time but the last six months felt different. I was more tired than usual. It was hard to point to a single symptom but something was off. Maybe it was time to slow down. With over a year of concert dates scheduled and a new album to record, it was hard to envision how to taper down.

I arrived at the studio and mustered the energy to walk up a short flight of stairs. It was strange to feel so depleted. I was a lifelong athlete and yogini. What was this about? Slowly laboring my way toward the entry, I felt progressively dizzier until everything went dark. It was the sound of the engineer calling my name that brought me back to consciousness.

The paramedics arrived in a flurry of efficiency. In seconds I had EEG monitors on my chest and back and a battery of basic tests were underway. My blood pressure, temperature, and heart rate were normal. Did I want to go to an emergency room for further tests? No, I was fine. I completed the recording session then called Lisa to let her know what happened. I didn't want to alarm her and I also knew that more than anyone, she was aware of my steady health decline. I couldn't pretend anymore.

Three days after this fainting episode, multiple blood tests and ultrasounds later, I was diagnosed with ovarian cancer. It would take another week before we discovered the innumerable pulmonary embolisms and blood clots. Part of the mystery was solved. We knew why I was feeling so bad. But the larger question remained, "What was it here to teach me?"

I found my first guidance in the poetry of the thirteenth century mystic poet, Rumi: "Find the antidote in the venom."

Because of the prevalence of cancer in our culture there are plenty of associated story lines. In researching possible treatments, I learned that although fairly rare, ovarian cancer is alarmingly lethal, killing two thirds of women diagnosed. In my condition, the innumerable pulmonary embolisms made the situation even more tenuous. Doctors gave me a 3% chance of survival. Everywhere I looked, I came upon the terms "war on cancer" or "the battle on cancer." What I knew from the start was that my body would not be a battleground. In order to heal I had to operate from wholeness and find connections instead of perpetuating a sense of separation and conflict.

The discovery of cancer in my body was like waking up and finding my basement flooded. As important as pumping out water and drying my furniture and belongings, the flooding water was a symptom of broken pipes I hadn't yet discovered. The "inconvenience" or "disturbance" of the flooded basement made me pay attention to something unseen that needed mending. My first step in healing was to understand this circumstance as an opportunity for growth and evolution. This cancer didn't happen "to" me. It happened "for" me. In order to fully recover from this serious health imbalance, I had to explore the deepest layers of my being.

Beneath the ego, beneath the personality, beneath the desires and fears, beneath the relationships, the traumas and victories, there is a stillness and intelligence that beckoned me closer. Because my body was so sick and my physical condition so compromised, I had to experience my "self" in a way that existed beyond the physical. My lungs and abdomen were filled with fluid and my once athletic and muscular legs had swollen beyond recognition making the simplest movements challenging. Every breath was a struggle. I needed a wheelchair to move.

Lying in the hospital bed, I found solace in gratitude. In the dark of a sleepless night, I slowly and methodically gave thanks. I was grateful for the steadiness of the floor beneath my hospital bed, grateful for the firmness of my teeth, the skin that wrapped my body, the faithfulness of my steady heart. Though each breath was a struggle, I was grateful for the abundance of nourishing air, grateful for the trees that helped produce it, grateful for the soil that nourished the trees. As my attention focused on the preponderance of good, it became easier to perceive this shift in my experience as part of a greater arc of goodness.

I wasn't afraid of dying as much as I felt like there was more for me to experience and learn in this physical form. As I wrote in my journal, "It's not a battle or a game to be won or lost. Each of us is going to die. The question is simply: How do we live? How do we bring the fullness of our being to every moment? Have we brought more love to those around us? It's not about errors, but about opportunities to adapt and evolve, to grow in awareness and become better human beings. My aim is to regain my health fully and be able to love more completely. If I have two years or fifty more, my prayer is: "May I live each day as fully as possible, love more abundantly, and leave the world a better place than I found it."

So the questions remained: "Why ovarian cancer?" and "Why now?"

I have always been drawn to music, poetry, and art because they express the language of the heart. They convey feelings that hover beyond the neat confines of measured speech. And being a lover of words who delights in speaking different languages, I also know the places where words are inadequate. I'm fascinated by science and math because they describe nature in a language that satisfies the mind. In answering these questions, I drew from these wells to develop metaphors and language which would guide my journey of discovery and healing.

Cancer is a chaotic proliferation of cells that do not serve the whole. They have no coherent relationship to the cells around them. They take without giving. They consume without serving. Conversely, healthy cells engage in a dynamic and beneficial relationship with their surrounding environment. When cancer is present, there is a breakdown in relationship. I began there.

Once they were discovered, I asked the tumors directly what they were about. Where did they come from? What were they holding? While meditating, I posed the question and the answer was immediate: "despair" and "mistrust." I hadn't even considered that I was harboring those emotions. As a confident and determined optimist, I set on my life's path as an artist and musician—and had succeeded. I was surprised by the discovery, but as I sat with it I felt a trap door lift from my heart and uncover a deep well of unexpressed emotion. Despair and mistrust. I realized that I had spent my life believing that I was here to be an agent of good, to be an "ambassador of kindness," but I couldn't fully trust the world to reciprocate. I was here to do good and be kind, but I couldn't trust the world to be good or kind in return. An inevitable despair resulted from this imbalance. My primary identity came through my creative expression, so it was no surprise that this imbalance presented in the energetic, creative seat of my physical being—my ovaries.

Because of the severity of my illness, I was literally and figuratively brought to my knees. Unable to move and barely able to breathe, there was nothing to do but surrender and ask for help. So I did. The extraordinary wave of love, kindness, and generosity began. As soon as I let my community know what had happened, an unimaginable deluge of support poured into my life. Whereas previously I was reluctant to share my struggles, ask for help, or reveal any weakness, I now had no option. My survival depended on it. I asked and the response was beyond anything I could have imagined. There were prayers, meals, phone calls, paintings, songs, visits—myriad expressions of love and goodness. Every day Lisa would return from the post office with cards and letters (many of them with financial support). I was deeply humbled. I cried every day—tears of joy, tears of relief, tears of recognition that it was not the world that lacked goodness, kindness or support but that my own unconscious beliefs had kept me from experiencing that flow of good. The onset of these life threatening physical circumstances had given me an opportunity to heal a deeper energetic imbalance than simply cancer.

Find the antidote in the venom.

Once I began to experience the power of metaphor, I embraced it on all fronts. When I say "metaphor," I mean tapping into a language beyond the intellect, beyond words, a language of the soul, a language of spirit, a language of the heart. This new language gave me an opportunity to navigate unfamiliar and dangerous terrain by creating relationships within a new framework. I began to see the cancer and the resulting clots as fiery, albeit unwanted, teachers who were there to push me to my next stage of evolution. Because of the severity of the condition, there was no room for wavering. The invitation was simply this: evolve or die. It wasn't just a cold. My life depended on it. I couldn't approach this challenge as something temporary either—like going on a diet, losing ten or twenty pounds, and then blithely returning to my former way of being. In order to live I had to die to my previous way of being. I had to release ways of thinking and acting that no longer served me. I was getting an opportunity to reincarnate in this lifetime…without having to suffer through seventh grade again!

I had long found solace in the scientific principle that for any system to change it must go through a period of chaos. Chaos is an essential quality in a thriving and ever evolving natural world. As any system grows or evolves it reaches a tipping point where it moves beyond predictability and becomes chaotic. At this point, it either collapses or reorders at a higher level of functioning. I began to see this episode with cancer as an opportunity for profound transformation and evolution, a chance to reorder at a higher level of functioning. How to do this?

First, every familiar pattern and rhythm was now in question. Because of my physical challenges, I couldn't get up and move and "do" things in the same way I had always done. I had to consciously rebuild the foundation of my life. Curiously, the house across the street was being completely renovated with carpenters, builders, and painters busily at work. As I lay in bed hearing the construction outside, I imagined that same level of renovation occurring internally—beginning with my consciousness and then filtering into my physical form.

Every moment was an opportunity to align with love, to remember my divine provenance. Though unable to move, I could still radiate love. Disconnected from my former life, I could still experience an unwavering connection to the sacred.

I imagined a caterpillar encased in her cocoon, entirely liquefying, and then emerging a butterfly. Transformation required a release of what had been. Curiously, as I lost all the hair on my head as a result of the chemotherapy and eventually, even my eyebrows, eyelashes, and the hair inside my nose, I felt I was returning to a near fetal state. This was the closest I had ever been to when my body took its first breath. I had never seen the curve of my bare scalp or the naked outlines of my eyelids. Rather than resisting this state I saw it as profound evidence of my renewal, my rebirth.

The mind is a powerful instrument of consciousness. It excels at organizing and analyzing information, and strategizing for outcomes with which it is already familiar. Meanwhile, the nature of life is constant change and expansion. There is an underlying pull to evolve. When we resist that evolution, our mind invariably comes up with a thousand excuses to remain on familiar ground. Growth, however, demands a departure from the predictable, from the known. When we lead from the heart and let love guide, we see a new and greater picture, a perfection of relationships and interaction that puts chaos and challenge into perspective. We begin to see obstacles as part of an inherent pull toward growth and expansion. Fear and resistance fall away.

My return to health meant understanding my "self" as more than just a physical expression. Healing my body meant healing the emotional/energetic layers as well as the physical. I underwent surgery and chemotherapy to eliminate the cancer. I shifted my diet and took high grade nutritional supplements. Even when I was physically unable to do my yoga practice, I would close my eyes and visualize an entire yoga session. I meditated. I exercised. I envisioned healing light coursing through my body. I released the parts of me that needed to be released.

Ideas, behaviors, and relationships that thwarted my authentic expression shifted in order for me to live. I engaged every aspect of my awareness to usher in the transformation required for my survival.

Nearly three years later, I am in remission and see this experience as a powerful and curious blessing. I occasionally come across pictures of myself as I was healing and it's hard to fathom the fragility and strength required to emerge from that dangerous encounter. At this point, I only have gratitude for the gifts I received along the journey. From the inside out, my life and sense of self have transformed. ♦

Divatude: Beauty in Spite of a Diagnosis—Daphne E.

"We regret to tell you, but you have been diagnosed with ovarian cancer." Those words changed my life and my aspect of life.

As a woman of curves, who believes in the "Female Form Divine" (Walt Whitman), I had finally learned to embrace the dip and sway of my body—the pure sensuality of being a woman, to make my curves work to my advantage. But it was not always so.

You see, I was one of those little girls who the kids used to make fun of because I had a little more padding; even my sisters would cajole me. From age six, I was always dieting or exercising. I even began weight training and it became an obsession.

But in 1998, at this diagnosis, I was shocked. Here I was in the best shape of my life: meeting body builders from WWE at Gold's Gym with my husband in Florida where I was inspired to really push my body to where I wanted it to be.

The surgeons said I would have to have a hysterectomy and at that time, I was thirty-five, married, and longing to have a child. The idea of losing a major part of my womanhood plunged me into despair. My marriage dissolved and I decided to start over and moved to San Francisco.

Even though I was still fighting, I became one of those career women overachievers. I had lost so much weight with the cancer that I was about a size three—and I felt that I was at my most attractive because I was finally thin. But as I look back, I was very sickly with body dysmorphia. Years later, I wrote this poem about my life's journey.

The Fat Girl

Tears streamed down my cheeks
As I ran up the drive,
Hearing shouts of "Boogley!"
From a busload of derisive children.
I heard the bus coming, I tried to escape them,
My legs betrayed me as I ran,
Refusing to help me.
They never saw my heart,
Hidden behind that eleven year old's chubby layer,
A heart breaking of being The Fat Girl.
My sisters laughed along,
Slim vixens they were,
I loved them, yet at times despised them,
Their thin waists taunted me.
I always prayed as I climbed on the scale,
"What are you today, a thousand and one?"
I cried when they laughed,
"God doesn't like ugly," I would say.
I dieted at age six,
Became anorexic at age fifteen,
Some days I thought I had won the battle,
Just to say that I had lost.
But one day cancer came to me,
It cleared my heart and mind
As it took away my weight.
It made me see how affected I was.
I forgave myself, I forgave my sisters,
I remembered that busload, I forgave those children.
Thank you God for helping me,
For in the mirror I now see a woman who loves who she is, A
Healthy Girl. ♦

(Printed with permission. ©2007 Daphne D. Evans)

After receiving a "cancer free" diagnosis in 2004, I went to Italy to celebrate. What I have found out is that during our cancer journey, when we are in remission, we must do something that we may have never tried before: get out and live!

So I went to Italy, very weak and tired, with a group of strangers. I had the time of my life. The tour guide couldn't understand why I would stay in bed some days. Finally I told him of my condition (not to gain pity, but boy, he was harsh!). His mannerism changed; he began to take me by the hand and make others walk ahead, saying, "Come little one." After coming home, I delved back into the world of hi-tech industry and law.

In 2005, because my back was hurting from the weight of my breasts (I was a DDD at only 4'11"), I decided to have a breast reduction. When I went in to see the doctor before the procedure, I had my first mammogram. A few days later, I received news that again brought me to my knees: there was a mass on my left breast. The ovarian cancer had metastasized as what is defined as "floaters" and had attached to my breast. So instead of a reduction, I had a double mastectomy.

I remember it clearly: I came home that day by myself, bandaged so tightly that my DDD chest was now flat as a board. I could not get past the mirrored armoire in the hallway. I stood there for countless minutes sobbing. I couldn't look myself in the eyes.

Angry and depressed, I asked God, "Why is this happening to me? Don't you think I've gone through enough?"

But the next day, I awoke with this peace of quiet resolve and what I was going to do about this. What would make me feel womanly again—full of sensuality and joie de vivre? One activity I always loved was going to the spa. So I went that day and received massage treatments. Well, it was so wonderful that I went for an entire week! That's when I made a choice.

I wasn't going to let cancer define me or allow it to rob me of feeling beautiful and creating joyous experiences.

I began to dress more stylishly—stilettos became my friend. I had regular appointments to get my hair and nails done, even going to get eyelash extensions when mine began to fall out. I bought higher count linens for my bed and spritzed them down with English lavender linen water before bedtime. One day I went to a high-end shop and bought all black lace lingerie! My gowns I wore for bed were 1930s vintage that I found on eBay—sensual and silky to the touch. I finally learned to put myself at the top of my priority list. I even coined a word for my new perspective: Divatude.

After the mastectomy (and my epiphany), I wanted other women to feel as beautiful as I did. That's why I began Heaven's Door Cancer Foundation that same year.

Heaven's Door is a wellness spa treatment and advocacy program for women with cancer and advanced life-threatening illnesses. Our purpose is Diva Aftercare: providing free spa visits for women going through cancer to maintain their inner fortitude and self-esteem. We send women to spas and resorts all across the U.S. I encourage my sisters (or "my divas") to feel beautiful despite the diagnosis.

But my battle with this disease continued.

In 2009, I was diagnosed with a third form of cancer: spinal. This one took me to a place of despair; my fiancé had passed away from colon cancer in 2008 and I refused to help myself. Help others yes, but me? No. I was tired and had no more will to live. I felt this big C was following wherever I went, even following the people I loved.

So I sold all of my things and moved to Springfield, MO, knowing only one person there. I found an old colonial home and renovated it, asking the interior design students of Missouri State University to take each room downstairs and remodel it. News channels begin to hear of my work and came with camera crews to record the renovation, including a dedicated massage and spa area. I wanted this to be my legacy, something that would continue on after I was gone.

Meanwhile, I would be in bed, sometimes for days at a time. My doctors had me on morphine to help with the pain. My brother came to help me; at night he would hear me crying. He would knock and when he wouldn't hear any answer, he would open the door, and see that I was trying to fall asleep, sobbing from the pain.

But the day came that the pain was so intense and my melancholy so overwhelming, I decided that there was no reason to prolong the pain. I decided to take my life. It was later determined that I took 21,000 milligrams of all of the meds that were given me and crushed them so that there was no way of turning back.

That day I remembered I could see the sun shining, but I felt as if I was looking from the bottom of a grave. I cried, asking God to forgive me, but I was so miserable and could no longer see the reason for living. My social worker called me and heard me crying. I asked her not to come, but she came and brought the ambulance. But coming to the ER, the doctors said because I had crushed them, there was not much they could do.

They gave me charcoal to drink and put me on renal failure watch.

As I lay there, I could see as if it were, a storm, billowing in the distance, coming closer and closer. Dark clouds, getting darker every minute. I knew it was death coming...then I heard a voice, saying, "Daphne, I'm here." It was the mother of my interior decorator. They had called her and she brought her mom. "I am going to pray for you. I am going to stand between you and death, because you have more work to do."

I whispered, "But the doctor said there is no hope."

She replied, "I don't care what they said. I will pray; you are going to be fine."

As she began to pray and I saw that darkness behind her, I began to cry, asking God to forgive me for trying to give back a gift that was given to me: the gift of life. I felt that a burden was being removed from me. I began to relax and heard her say that she had to leave, but she knew I would be okay.

That night the doctors told me that all of the poison went past my kidneys, through my digestive system, and that I should be dead. That is when I knew that God was with me and not allowing me to die for a reason. It gave me the strength to fight not only death and cancer, but to get better.

I began going to church where this kind lady who prayed for me (who I called Mama) and her husband led a "coffee house" church at their home. It was very relaxing and a small group. They would come pick me up from my house and take me there.

Sometimes the pain was so terrific that I would have to lie down or walk around, but I still went. One day in the middle of the pain, I asked them if they would do the old-fashioned thing and put me in a chair, surround me, and pray for me. I knew I would have to make the decision to go into surgery and I was afraid. Being a kid growing up in church, my parents had done this before to those who were infirmed. I didn't want any hocus pocus now, just a quiet prayer in giving this situation over to God. I even asked them to find some oil like they used back in the Bible to anoint one's head and pray. I was pulling out the stops. What harm could it do? So they did, and they all begin to pray that God's will be done in my life.

I sat there quietly absorbing all of the positive energy surrounding me. Then I felt something that touched the top of my head and traveled in lightning speed down my spine. Now, I am very down to earth and believed in such things, but not to the extent that something like that would happen in this day and age. I was a believer, but not to the place of this. But what happened was that Mama felt it, too, and she jumped back as if she had been shocked by electricity. We looked at each other asking, "Did you feel that?" No one else felt it but us.

She asked me if I felt differently. I told her that, truthfully, my back still ached, but maybe not as bad. I wasn't going to commit to a miracle. To me? No way.

But going to my doctor's office, she said that though I felt better, my pain level had increased my blood pressure to 210/120 and I was the verge of a stroke. I had to make the decision for them to start working to remove this tumor. Nothing more could be done until I gave them the go ahead.

So again, I went back to my little prayer group that Sunday and asked that they would pray that God would give me the courage to go through one more surgery, that my spine would not be severed. They all began to pray again, one after the other. So many tears and prayers that in some way, God would be glorified in this horrible situation. I sat there with my head bowed, feeling peace come over me as if I could feel a palpable spirit of quietness and peace standing there.

That Monday I went in for my first step—an MRI which would show them exactly where the tumor was. Then they would shoot it full of anesthesia to freeze it and then try to remove it. When I went into radiology that day, the technician had this placard on her desk: "And it shall come to pass that before they call, I will answer; while they are yet speaking, I will hear." Isaiah 65:24.

I took that with me as I lay in that chamber, asking God to give me the strength to go through one more surgery, that all of my other cancers were surgically removed and I believed He would help me get through this one more test.

On Wednesday, they called me with the results and our plan of procedure. The doctor sounded a little strange. "Daphne, I called to give you the results of the MRI. The tumor is gone." I nearly fell to the ground. "What...what?"

"Yes, we see where it was because you have substantial nerve damage there, but it is as if it was just removed. Now, we know these things can happen, but as scientists we cannot explain how."

"Did you look everywhere? You know how I have floating mets."

"Yes, we have done an extensive search and it is nowhere to be found. We need you to continue on a pain management course and start with physical therapy, but you will no longer need surgery."

When I hung up, I was standing in my backyard. I began to dance, crying, "Thank you my Father God! (Ouch, ouch!) Thank you for removing this from my body!" I ran to the computer and I went to Facebook and posted my report and my friends from all over the country began to celebrate with me.

Many who weren't even believers as I was said how they had actually prayed and sent positive vibes and good thoughts my way. Hundreds had been raising me up and I didn't even know. I thought because I had left San Francisco that I had been forgotten. But they were still holding me in their hearts.

After that I decided to get off every medicine and pain pill they had me on; yes, I was still in pain, but if God brought me this far, I believed that I would be okay.

My dear Mama came to me. "Honey, I think you should give up the house and come and be with us and let us help you through this."

I was so fiercely independent that at first I said no. Then I heard this clearly, "It takes grace to give, but graciousness to receive."

I could not run a cancer foundation until I myself was healthy.

So they moved me and my two doggies into one of the wings of their huge beautiful home (when God blesses you, it is never less than the best!) and began to go through detox. From lemon infusions to organic eating with prayer and meditation every morning and evening.

Slowly walking the grounds of their beautiful ranch, and going to gather the hen's eggs from the hen house, I began to receive clarity of spirit and heart and body. I would wake up in the middle of the night with bursts of joy and thanking God for His blessing of life and happiness.

Within a month and a half, I was off every pill and pain free. Yes, pain free.

I stayed in Missouri for another six months and then knew I must return to the work I was called to do: to help my sisters in any way I can during their fight with cancer.

I came back to San Francisco to continue Heaven's Door Cancer Foundation. Not to get back to status quo—working sixty-hour weeks to have the fine mansion and the fancy car—but to work enough days to pay my bills and the rest of the time be dedicated to my ladies.

Our mission is to assist those with advanced life-threatening illness, to maintain dignity, function, and a high quality of life throughout their course of illness. We will help women undergoing treatments such as surgery, chemo, or radiation cope with the emotionally traumatic and emotional side effects of treatment. I will go with them to the hospitals and be waiting in recovery when they come out of surgery. To be with them during hospice and even speak at their funerals. These are my sisters, my family.

My main objective is to help my divas regain a sense of self confidence and control over their lives and advanced life-threatening illnesses. I have written poetry, spoken at conferences, been on tv, been interviewed by Ebony, Jet, Essence as well as other national magazines. We host fashion show fundraisers and different holiday events to raise money to take care of women: ranging from those who are even pregnant and dealing with cancer and chemotherapy to women who are in hospice centers needing pampering and attention.

This year I am taking four single moms battling cancer to Hawaii for a vacation.

Right now, I thank God that all of my cancers are still in remission.

My message to my sisters is this: Yes, you have cancer, your head is bald from the chemo, and you feel sick a lot of the time. But when you're what I call a cancer diva, you don't have to take any of it lying down. There's still so much to celebrate...starting with the fact that you're here.

Finally, I have been working with so many women dealing with breast cancer and having a hard time with the mastectomy side of it.

Quite a few of these ladies are like me who had "big beautiful ones" and the identity crisis is hitting them hard. I decided to write a poem regarding our struggle. This is dedicated to all women who have gone through so much and will not give up.

The Breastplate of Beauty

You look down,
Curves so familiar, so comforting,
They started young, got you noticed,
Blushing when the boys pointed,
Pulling out your sweater to try to hide them.
But they were yours and they were beautiful,
They were a part of you.
They grew with you,
Drove you crazy when trying to contain them,
Stretching your aching back when you carried them,
But you would give them up for nothing.
They were a part of you.
You dreamed of motherhood,
Again looking down,
Seeing the peaceful face of a child
Sweet, innocent tulip mouth in the natural state of supping
Smiling, you held them close to you,
Wonderful nurturer that you are.
But now you must say good bye with tears in your eyes,
Saying "Farewell" to the gifts God has bestowed on every woman,
They did not define you as a person,
but They were a part of you.
Look up, woman warrior!
Let your battle scars become your breastplate of beauty,
Learn to stand tall again,
straighten those shoulders that once held the weight,
A weight that is no longer there.
Look at yourself in the mirror,
And say, I am a beautiful warrior!
I have survived the battle and have overcome the war.
For though they are gone, I am alive! And though they were a part
of me, I AM STILL ME. ♦

(Printed with permission. ©2013 Daphne D. Evans)

CHAPTER 23
DIABETES

Plenty of people have proven that the
right diet reverses type 2 diabetes.

Have you recently consumed a snack or meal high in carbohydrates or sugar without added protein? You've just generated a rapid rise in your blood glucose. We all need a certain amount of carbs. However, through our addiction to refined, processed foods and sweets, diabetes has become the fastest growing disease in our country. Pre-diabetes cases are also rapidly rising.

Diabetes is a chronic health condition traditionally characterized by elevated levels of glucose in your blood, or simply put, high blood sugar. Type 2 diabetes makes up 90% of diabetes cases.

The World Health Organization (WHO) expects 300 million cases worldwide by 2025. Sadly, overweight children and adolescents are being diagnosed at an alarming rate. One in three Americans, including children, will contract diabetes. Among minorities, the rate will be one in two.

What Causes Diabetes?

Diabetes is caused by genetics, lifestyle, and environmental factors. The worldwide epidemic of type 2 diabetes can be attributed to the standard American diet (SAD) with its emphasis on consuming refined and processed carbohydrates, fructose, high fructose corn syrup, high sugar intake, and lack of exercise. There are three main types of diabetes:

1. **Type 1 diabetes.** Insulin Dependent. This form often affects children, but adults can develop it, too. In this form of diabetes, the body can't make insulin. The immune system, by mistake, attacks

the cells in the pancreas that make and release insulin. As these cells die, blood sugar levels rise. People with type 1 diabetes need insulin shots.

2. **Type 2 diabetes.** Largely Non-Insulin Dependent. People with type 2 diabetes can't maintain normal blood sugar levels. This happens either because the body doesn't make enough insulin or because the body can't use its own natural insulin properly—a process called insulin resistance. When people are insulin resistant, their muscle, fat, and liver cells do not respond properly to insulin. As a result, their bodies need more insulin to help glucose enter cells.

Glucose is created when your body breaks down food to use for energy. Your body uses glucose as its main source of fuel with the help of the hormone insulin. Insulin acts like a key to unlock the body's cells, so glucose can enter and serve as fuel for the cells. The pancreas tries to keep up with this increased demand but eventually fails. Excess glucose builds up in the bloodstream, setting the stage for diabetes.

3. **Gestational diabetes.** This type of diabetes occurs in some pregnant women. It can cause problems during pregnancy, labor, and delivery. Women who get gestational diabetes are more likely to develop type 2 diabetes.

Diabetes is not a disease to ignore as it can rob you of many years of healthy living. Early detection of diabetes decreases the chance of developing complications. An overall healthy diet and lifestyle can stabilize your blood sugar and reverse adult-onset diabetes.

In a report published in *The New England Journal of Medicine*, Walter Willett, MD, PhD, from the Harvard School of Public Health demonstrated that 91% of all type 2 diabetes could be prevented through aggressive changes in diet and lifestyle. Following is a story that illustrates this point.

How I Manage Diabetes—Janice C.

I have always loved sweets, and now my poor habits have caught up with me. My blood sugar has always been in the normal range and besides my love of sweets, I eat a pretty healthy diet and do a moderate exercise routine.

When my blood sugar level went up my doctor recommended that I take medication. I first wanted to see if lifestyle changes would lower my blood sugar. I was quite anxious about this but my doctor agreed to let me try exercising more and avoiding sugar and junk food (food not in its natural state).

To help balance my blood sugar, my doctor recommended that I make exercise a priority. At the same time, I gave up white flour, sugar, and processed foods that made my blood glucose spike. Changing my sugar habit was the hardest part, even though I knew it was bad for my body and my skin.

Instead of sweets, I now eat delicious snacks such as hummus and homemade guacamole or apple with almond butter. When other people are eating foods full of sugar like cakes, cookies, and ice cream, I indulge in dark chocolate or other desserts sweetened with Stevia or Xylitol. Dessert is only a momentary pleasure. You eat it and it's done. What lasts is the good feeling I get from seeing healthier numbers on my blood work. As a result, I've avoided going on medication for my diabetes. ♦

Below is Kathy's story of how she avoided going on medication for diabetes.

Taking Diabetes into My Own Hands—Kathy B.

When I got diagnosed with type 2 diabetes and learned that my blood glucose was more than double the normal level, I got really worried. One of my older siblings had diabetes and I didn't want to follow in his footsteps, depending on pills and eventually insulin.

I did research online, read books on diabetes, and immediately began eating differently. I started with making green smoothies with green leafy vegetables, green apple, protein powder, and flaxseed for breakfast. I cut out sweets, cut back on carbs, and added lots of salads and steamed vegetables. I can eat big portions of these foods so I don't feel deprived in any way. I also joined a health club and began taking exercise classes.

Reversing diabetes required commitment on my part, but I have no desire to return to my old habits. My taste buds won't accept poor quality food anymore. I'm used to really nutritious food now and I feel younger than ever. ♦

How I Managed Gestational Diabetes—Alice Z., MD

When I was pregnant with my first child, my sugar was high normal and I did not pay attention to my diet. I ended up with an eight-pound baby and had a third-degree tear during delivery that required blood transfusion. It was not fun.

In my second pregnancy I was diagnosed with glucose intolerance and had to work on my diet. I did and had a normal delivery.

When I was pregnant with my third child, I gained a lot of weight in the first trimester, and was diagnosed with gestational diabetes. I had been feeling thirsty and extremely exhausted with this pregnancy. I felt that I could fall asleep while driving back home from work.

When I got that diagnoses from my OB/GYN doctor I said to myself, "That can't be true." I wanted to retest it.

As a physician I'd been treating patients with diabetes. I thought, "I can't have diabetes myself." I was in denial, partially because I was well aware what diabetes involves.

I finally admitted to having diabetes. I didn't want a big baby resulting from diabetes or trouble with my delivery. I saw the diabetes nurse and began checking blood sugar levels four times a day by pricking my finger, and started to follow the diet she gave me.

The nurse would review my sugar levels and give me recommendations on how to change my diet. I prepare my own lunch most of the time and if I eat at a lunch meeting, I also count the carbs to make sure I don't overeat. If it is a big meal, I save some for a snack at a later time. In the morning, I can't drink milk because it is considered high carb which can make sugar high. In the morning, the pregnancy hormone is highest so I had to limit the carbs to only small servings. I noticed I cannot eat white rice and noodles like I used to because it spikes my sugar levels over 200. Instead I eat plain yogurt with fruit or nuts as my snack.

It was a lot of work to count the carbs and prepare my meals. Sometimes when the kids were eating yummy cakes or cookies it was hard to resist because I have a sweet tooth. I resisted most of the time, and the sugar number was usually good, so I didn't have to take medicine or shoot insulin.

One day I was driving to work and realized I felt cool and calm without the sweaty feeling I often had after eating milk and bread for breakfast. Also, when I was driving back home from work I noticed I was very alert and energized. I used to almost dose off when I drove home before I changed my diet. Wow! I said to myself, this diet not only brings the sugar number down, but also makes me feel energized. I like that! This was the first time I realized that the food we are eating can change the way our body feels. What a powerful thing. It was a lot of work but it was definitely worth all the effort. I have three healthy children and I am happy to say I no longer have diabetes.

This is what my diet was like before and after being diagnosed with diabetes.

Breakfast: I used to eat waffles, bread, or pancakes and a glass of milk. I switched to one piece of sprouted grain bread or bagel, an egg, and tea.

Mid-morning: I have a cup of yogurt with fruit.

Lunch: I eat a small amount of brown rice with stir fried veggies and some chicken or pork. At work we also have meetings with a free lunch. In this case I eat one small sandwich with water or tea, or only one slice of pizza with some salad. For Mexican type of lunch, I have to leave out either the beans or the rice because it's too many carbs. For a Chinese boxed lunch, I only eat half of the white rice.

Mid-afternoon: Around 3:30 p.m. I eat some nuts and plain yogurt or fruit again.

Dinner: I eat with my family, and we changed from white rice to brown rice. We always have fish, chicken, or pork, and sautéed or stir-fried veggies. I only eat a small portion of brown rice, noodles, or dumplings. I read labels and count the servings of carbs for each snack and meal. ♦

A Few Words about Carbs—Sheri M.

Many sources, including the Diabetes Association, suggest forty-five to sixty grams of carbohydrates per meal for diabetics. Some people do well with carbs. What I notice is that if I have more than about fifteen carbs per meal, I may get sleepy and sluggish. I find I feel best including protein at every meal and minimizing carbohydrates.

Each person must determine the number of carbs per meal that they feel best on. ♦

Symptoms of Type 2 Diabetes

Some of the symptoms of diabetes may easily be overlooked but may indicate a pre-diabetic condition. What are the symptoms of type 2 diabetes? The symptoms vary from person to person but may include:

- Increased thirst
- Increased hunger (especially after eating)
- Frequent urination
- Fatigue (weak, tired feeling)
- Blurred vision
- Numbness or tingling of the hands or feet

How Do Doctors Diagnose Diabetes?

1. If your blood glucose level is 200 milligrams per deciliter, regardless of the time of day you are fasting, or

2. Two separate blood tests show that your fasting blood glucose level is 126 mg/dl (7.0 mmol/l) or higher after an 8-hour fast, or

3. In some cases, doctors perform a glucose tolerance test. If your blood glucose value is 200 mg/d (11.1 mmol/l0) or higher two hours later a doctor will diagnose diabetes.

Diabetes, Leptin, and Insulin Resistance

Leptin is a hormone produced in your fat cells. One of its primary roles is to regulate your appetite and body weight. It tells your brain when to eat, how much to eat, and when to stop eating, which is why it's called the "satiety hormone." It also tells your brain what to do with the energy it has. Leptin is responsible for the accuracy of insulin signaling and for your insulin resistance.

A primary role of insulin is not to lower your blood sugar, but to store the extra energy for future consumption. According to Dr. Ron Rosedale, chief medical officer at Advanced Medical Labs, University of Colorado, states, "Diabetes is not a disease of blood sugar, but rather a disorder of insulin and leptin signaling." Elevated insulin levels are not only symptoms of diabetes, but also heart disease, peripheral vascular disease, stroke, high blood pressure, cancer, and obesity.

The only known way to reestablish proper leptin and insulin signaling is through your diet. This can have a more profound influence on your health than any known drug or modality of medical treatment.

Serious Health Consequences

Over time, high levels of glucose in the blood can harm your whole body. Type 2 diabetes can lead to dangerous health problems and can include:

- stroke
- eye problems including glaucoma or blindness

- hearing loss
- high blood pressure
- heart disease
- gum disease
- nerve damage which can lead to problems requiring amputation of lower limbs
- kidney disease, sometimes serious enough to require an organ transplant
- foot problems, such as infections and sores

Diabesity

Diabesity is both preventable and reversible by lifestyle choices.
—Mark Hyman, MD

Mark Hyman, MD, is the author of five best-selling books. His most recent is *The Blood Sugar Solution*. Dr. Hyman coined the term "diabesity" to describe what he calls the "hidden time bomb of disease that lies at the root of aging, weight gain, and today's most prevalent chronic conditions." Diabesity is a combination of health problems ranging from mild insulin resistance and overweight, to obesity and diabetes. Symptoms may include weight gain around the belly, and swings in blood pressure that make you feel anxious, irritable, or tired, and can even cause palpitations and panic attacks.

Dr. Hyman blames the standard American diet (SAD) as the leading cause of diabesity. Too many refined, sugary carbohydrates and beverages trigger insulin resistance. Insulin resistance occurs when cells slowly become resistant—or numb—to the effects of insulin and need more and more of it to keep blood sugar levels balanced. A high insulin level is the first sign, but most doctors never test this. Rather, they test blood sugar levels, but these rise above healthy levels only after insulin has been elevated for some time.

Insulin from excess carbohydrates promotes fat and then wards off the body's ability to lose that fat. The way to protect your body from storing fat and rising insulin levels is through reducing refined carbs and eliminating sugars from your diet. Several studies conducted over the past decade have demonstrated that reduction in carbohydrates leads to weight loss and improved blood sugars in people with diabetes.

Dr. Hyman recommends testing of insulin levels for anyone who has a family history of type 2 diabetes, belly fat or increased waist size, or abnormal cholesterol.

According to Dr. Hyman, the key to overcoming diabesity is not to focus on lowering blood sugar by taking medications but rather to focus on diet, exercise and lifestyle. He states that "cutting out or drastically reducing starches and sugars and exercising" is the cure for most people.

Important Guidelines for Reversing or Preventing Diabetes

- Eat snacks and meals that include protein and healthy fats every three to four hours.
- Reduce sugar intake and find a sugar alternative such as stevia or xylitol you enjoy that does not spike blood sugar. See more ideas in the chapter on sugar.
- Eat an abundance of non-starchy vegetables. Examples: kale, collard greens, chard, asparagus, broccoli, cauliflower, spinach, tomatoes, celery, cabbage, carrots, sweet peppers, green beans, sprouts, and cucumbers.
- Eat limited quantities of whole, unrefined grain. Choose those high in fiber such as: brown rice, quinoa, oatmeal, buckwheat, and millet. Whole grains contain both magnesium and chromium, along with fiber, which helps to slow digestion and control blood sugar levels. Whole grains take longer to digest than refined breads, pasta, sugary breakfast cereal, cookies, or pastry.
- Limit fruit intake to one or two portions a day. Buy organic when possible. (Dried fruits are much higher in sugar as well as tropical fruits like pineapple and mango.)

- Choose healthy fats like those found in olive oil, avocado, nuts, seeds, flax, and oily fish like salmon and sardines.
- Eat healthy protein sources such as lean meat, beans, legumes, nuts, and seeds. Avoid peanuts due to their high mold content which produces aflatoxin, a carcinogen.
- Eat fish two or three times a week, choosing kinds that are high in heart-protective fat and low in mercury (such as salmon, sardines, and herring).
- Limit your intake of salt and sodium.
- Keep healthy snacks on hand so you don't have to resort to junk food or fast food. Examples: apple slices with almond butter, handful of nuts or seeds, boiled egg, hummus and whole grain crackers, yogurt, kefir, or goat cheese. Eat dairy in limited quantities.
- Avoid sugary drinks/trans fats/nitrates. Fast food and packaged foods frequently contain trans fats (also known as hydrogenated oil) which increase inflammatory processes associated with diabetes.
- Manage your weight. Eating a healthy diet and incorporating more activity into your life will help you achieve this goal.
- De-stress. Lowering stress is especially important for people with diabetes. When you're stressed, glucose levels can spike. To keep stress at bay, take time to simply breathe deeply and quiet your mind. See final chapter for more ideas to relax and de-stress.
- Get moving. Aim for thirty minutes of physical activity most days of the week. Physical activity lowers your blood sugar. It boosts your energy, relieves stress, and reduces your risk of heart disease and stroke. Find activities you enjoy. Consider dancing, a workout DVD, or taking a brisk walk with family, friends, or your furry friend.
- Compose a healthy meal. Composing a healthy meal is an essential life skill. Here's an easy way to make over your diet.

Draw an imaginary line down the middle of your plate and fill half of your plate with non-starchy vegetables (such as salad, spinach, broccoli, asparagus, kale, or green beans) using a healthy fat such as olive oil. Divide the other side of your plate in half and fill one quarter section with healthy protein such as lean meat or fish. Fill the last quarter section with whole grains such as brown rice, quinoa, or a starchy vegetable such as carrots, peas or potatoes.

In addition to the guidelines listed above, here is a list of supplements that can help slash your risk of diabetes:

1. **Magnesium.** This mineral helps promote healthy insulin production. A magnesium rich diet has been shown to lower risks.

2. **Alpha-lipoic Acid.** A fatty acid found naturally in the body and in small amounts in some foods, this powerful antioxidant neutralizes potentially harmful free radicals.

3. **Chromium.** If you're not taking diabetes medications you might consider a chromium supplement. Chromium can help to lower glucose levels as well as reduce belly fat, another risk factor. If you are on medication, consult your physician.

4. **Biotin.** Biotin has been shown to enhance insulin sensitivity, lower triglycerides, and improve glucose metabolism.

5. **Vitamin D3.** This supplement improves metabolism by influencing more than 200 different genes that can prevent and treat type 2 diabetes and metabolic syndrome. (Get your blood tested to determine your vitamin D levels.)

6. **Cinnamon and Green Tea.** Cinnamon and green tea are helpful in controlling blood sugar and improving insulin sensitivity. Green tea can even increase fat burning and metabolism.

7. **Protein Powder.** A high-quality protein powder in a smoothie can help balance your blood sugar and makes an excellent choice for breakfast or snack.

Diabetes Facts

- One of the most important dietary changes a diabetic can make is eliminating sugar (especially fructose) and limiting grains in the diet.
- Insulin regulation plays such an integral role in your health and longevity that elevated levels are not only symptoms of diabetes, but can also be indicators of heart disease, peripheral vascular disease, stroke, high blood pressure, cancer, and obesity.
- *The New England Journal of Medicine* has acknowledged the fact that diet and exercise can cure type 2 diabetes.
- High blood sugar can harm your organs and sets off processes that can lead to complications. Keeping your blood sugar balanced lowers your risk for multiple health problems down the road.
- There is a strong link between type 2 diabetes and obesity as it's more difficult for the cells to interact with insulin in a person who is also overweight.
- The way to reestablish proper leptin and insulin signaling is through your diet which can have a more profound influence on diabetes than any known drug or modality of medical treatment.

In Conclusion

Type 2 diabetes is one of the easiest diseases to overcome by making lifestyle changes. If you have diabetes, you already know you're living with a serious condition. What you may not realize is you are in the driver's seat. With healthy habits such as exercising and making smart food choices, you have the power to improve and reverse your diabetes. By doing so, you'll be doing yourself and those who depend on you a favor by adding years to your life.

CHAPTER 24
GOOD FATS, BAD FATS

Jack Sprat could eat no fat,
his wife could eat no lean;
And so between them both,
They licked the platter clean.

Fear of Eating Fat

You're not alone in your fear of eating fat. "Eat a low-fat, low-cholesterol diet" is a recommendation we've heard so often we can recite it in our sleep. Unfortunately, this message is out of date. A healthy diet is not a "fat–free" diet. Rather, our diet should consist of beneficial, good fats.

The main idea of this chapter is to learn how to substitute "bad" fats with "good" fats. An estimated 80% of Americans eat a diet deficient in omega-3 essential fatty acids (EFAs), which is especially unfortunate considering our bodies cannot make EFAs. The idea of eating fat to get healthier or to lose weight may be counter intuitive to everything you've heard about the dangers of fat. What really matters is the type of fat.

The Right Kind of Fat

Research shows that the right kind of fat stimulates the body's metabolic ability to burn fat. In Dr. Ann Louise Gittleman's book *The Fat Flush Plan*, that's exactly what she advocates. Gittleman is an award-winning *New York Times* bestselling author of thirty books on health and nutrition. Gittleman says that the right kind of fat will help you lose weight without being overly preoccupied with dieting and that essential fats are absolutely necessary for weight loss, longevity, and good health.

In Gloria's upcoming story, she demonstrates how consuming healthy fats can actually help you lose the weight you want, in her case, seventy pounds! She worked with The Fat Flush Plan that emphasizes consuming healthy fats as a key component to achieving one's ideal weight.

What Can Essential Fatty Acids (EFAs) Do for You?

Essential Fatty Acids (EFAs) help build cells, regulate the nervous system, strengthen the cardiovascular system, build immunity, and help the body absorb nutrients. EFAs are vital for healthy brain function and vision. After all, your brain is 60% fat. Every cell in your body is protected by a membrane that is composed largely of fat. With the right fats, you'll feel more full and satisfied, have more energy, and lose the weight you want.

The Vital Role of Good Fats

- Reducing inflammation
- Weight loss
- Cell communication
- Brain function
- Maintaining normal cholesterol levels
- Immune system function
- Building our energy reserves

Distinction between Omega-3 and Omega-6

There are two families of EFAs: omega-6 (linoleic acid) and omega-3 (alpha-linolenic acid). Omega-3s are plentiful in diets of unprocessed foods and where grazing animals eat grass. Omega-9 is healthy but not "essential" because the body makes it, unlike omega-3 and 6.

Today's Western diets are overloaded with omega-6s, mainly in refined vegetable oils from soybean, corn, and canola and from the meat of animals that are fed grain as opposed to grass. While oil coming from vegetables seems healthy, these are examples of oils that are refined and contribute to inflammation.

Refined vegetable oils that are used in most snack foods, cookies, crackers, and sweets are the major source of excess omega-6s in the average Western diet. Both omega-3 and omega-6 fats are polyunsaturated fatty acids (PUVAs) and they're both essential to your health, but when omega-6 is consumed *in excess*, it becomes problematic. When consumed in the wrong ratios, they tend to stimulate inflammatory processes in your body, rather than inhibit them.

Meeting Gloria—Angie L.

I met and interviewed Gloria after learning she had lost seventy pounds the good, old fashioned way through healthy eating and exercise. After reading several weight-loss books, Gloria's favorite was *The Fat Flush Plan* (TFFP) which emphasizes consuming healthy fats as a key component in this weight loss plan.

TFFP relies on the combination of healthy essential fats, protein, and colorful carbohydrates. Natural weapons for losing weight: 1. flaxseeds, 2. flaxseed oil, and 3. unsweetened cranberry juice. Flaxseeds fill you up, cleanse, and heal at the same time. Gloria's story demonstrates how healthy fats can help you lose the weight you want.

Eat Healthy Fats to Lose Weight—Gloria A.

In May of 2005, I didn't fit into a size eighteen anymore. At Macy's, when I couldn't zip up a pair of size eighteen pants, the sales clerk referred me to the plus size department. That's when I knew I'd let myself go for too long. I was addicted to carbs and considered myself the "queen of junk food." It was time for a change.

I started by reading dozens of books on nutrition, health, cleansing, and weight loss. After I decided to lose weight, I remember making the decision to clean out my pantry. I never realized how much junk food and processed food I consumed until I reevaluated my fridge and pantry. All the food lacked nutritious value and were loaded with sugar and carbs. I immediately threw everything into garbage bags and decided it was time to completely change my lifestyle. I made the conscious decision not to ever buy junk food again. I replaced it all with organic, raw food. Instead of buying dressings for the new food to give it flavor, I began making my own with olive oil and lemon.

I quit my lucrative sales job to focus on getting healthy and achieving my ideal weight.

After two months, I started losing ten pounds per month consistently. By the seventh month, I weighed sixty pounds less and lost an additional ten pounds a few months later.

My Diet: The first year I ate protein (salmon, tofu, and chicken) and all kinds of steamed vegetables. No sugar, dairy product, salt, salad dressing, or anything processed. Instead, I learned to use natural spices such as ginger, onion, garlic, cinnamon, parsley, paprika, lemon, lime, flaxseed oil, and cilantro to flavor my food. My favorite dessert was frozen fruit (blueberries). In my second year, I started eating barley, lentils, and beans. Now in my third year, I just introduced Organic Sprouted 100% Flourless Tortillas from Whole Foods and the brand is Fat Flush Plan (French Meadow Bakery).

I went from a plus size to a size two/four and now weigh 120 pounds.

My favorite book and best strategy for losing the weight? *The Fat Flush Plan* (TFFP). I consider it a great beginning book to make the transition from bad fats/high sugar/junk type foods to a truly healthy, nutritious diet. TFFP teaches natural, safe strategies that promote healthy weight loss and good health. There are three very distinct phases in TFFP.

If one desires to lose more than twenty-five pounds, one can safely remain on Phase I for up to one month. Phase I of the plan includes no wheat (and no starches), very little dairy, no sugar (this includes honey, agave, all forms of sugar) and no caffeine or alcohol.

Phase I is focused on drinking flaxseed/cranberry juice three to four times per day and eating tons of colored carbohydrates with a focus on lots of vegetables.

The first two weeks of Phase I is a true body cleanse. After completing Phase I, you move on to Phase II, which incorporates more foods, and eventually to Phase III.

My natural weapon for losing weight was the long-life cocktail made of flaxseeds and flaxseed oil, combined with unsweetened cranberry juice (okay to sweeten with Stevia). Flaxseeds and flaxseed oil fill you up, cleanse, and provide many health benefits at the same time.

My favorite flaxseed (after researching many) is made by Health From The Sun and is called FiProFLAX. It's organic, premium, cold pressed flaxseed. The flaxseed/cranberry drink curbs your carb and sugar cravings while allowing you to enjoy the health benefits of omegas.

Phase I (first two weeks) requires discipline, self-control, consistency, determination, and an understanding of how the body processes food. This knowledge can be obtained from Gittleman's book *The Fat Flush Plan*.

I strongly believe that if you want to make permanent changes, it has to be from the most natural state of food. I did not trust any weight loss plan that was not based on healthy food, healthy fats, and moderate exercise. The decision to take supplements is personal and up to each individual. I cannot overstate how important it is to reaffirm your goals and intentions each day to keep yourself motivated and on purpose.

One of my purposes for losing weight was a dream to one day hike the Incan mountains of my native country, Peru. I trained hard and accomplished my goal of hiking the 50-kilometer trek in June of the following year, 2006.

After eating this way for five years, I inspired my teenage daughter with the value of eating good food. She not only lost weight, but developed a healthy lifestyle. Even in college, she makes smart food decisions at her college's dining hall. Now, she wants to share her healthy eating tips with her friends and other young girls on her personal blog. ♦

Tips for Shifting Your Diet

1. To change and replace habits, you have to be ready. Good intentions are not enough. You have to have conviction, determination, self-control, and purpose.

2. Reaffirm your goals each day to keep yourself motivated and on purpose!

3. You are guaranteed increased vitality, energy, and happiness in addition to your personal goals by eating and living this new, healthy way.

4. Your environment is crucial. You need support from loved ones. Let them know your goals. Be firm.

5. Connect with people who are doing healthy things (walking groups, hiking groups, health club, running, spinning, tennis, and swimming.)

6. Portions at restaurants are often too big so split meals with friends or take half the meal home.

7. Do some form of cardio exercise thirty to forty-five minutes three to four times per week.

8. Learn to use the power of your mind to focus on achieving what you desire. Meditation and visualization are a good place to start.

9. Do things that make you feel good (listen to music, dance, meditate, yoga, tai chi).

10. Affirm the positives in your life: I am healthy. I am strong. I am successful.

EFA Imbalance Leads to Inflammation

Ideally the body's ratio of omega-3 to omega-6 should be in a range of 1:1. The problem? In today's modern American diet, it is estimated that omega-6 fatty acids dominate omega-3 by ratios ranging from 20:1 to 50:1. In other words, Americans currently consume between twenty and fifty times the healthy level of omega-6 fats to omega-3 fatty acids. These huge imbalances of omega-6 encourage chronic inflammation.

With omega-6 being pro-inflammatory when out of balance with omega-3, you can see why most Americans are dealing with some type of inflammation! This imbalance contributes to illnesses such as heart disease, type 2 diabetes, and other chronic diseases.

The Power of Omega-3 Essential Fatty Acids (EFAs)

The cardio-protective power of omega-3 has been thoroughly documented in clinical literature. Less well known is its paramount role in optimizing brain function.

Omega-3 fatty acids are the building blocks for an estimated 100 billion neurons and are our first-line supplement for preventing and reversing inflammation. Embedded in the omega-3 rich neuronal membrane are numerous proteins and complex molecules required for electrochemical transmission and signal reception.

Health Benefits of Omega-3

- Inhibits cancer
- Lowers blood pressure, platelet stickiness, and cardiovascular risk
- Normalizes fat metabolism in diabetes
- Causes weight loss by increasing metabolic rate and fat burn off
- Helps relieve arthritis inflammation
- Improves the condition of hair, nails, and skin
- Improves certain kinds of eczema
- Slows down or stops deterioration of MS
- Helps treat diabetic neuropathy in type 2 diabetes
- Kills cancer cells without harming normal cells (overabundance of omega-6 enhances tumor growth)
- Regulates every bodily function at the cellular level

Omega-3 and Omega-6 Food Sources

Omega-6 (Consume smaller amounts because most of us get too much of this type of fat.)

Food sources containing omega-6 include peanut oil, soybean oil, canola oil, walnut oil, sunflower oil, pumpkin seeds, corn oil, safflower oil, sesame oil, peanuts, pine nuts or snack foods containing these oils; margarine and shortening oils made with hydrogenated oils (trans fats), and corn-fed beef.

Omega-3 (Consume larger amounts because most of us could use more of this healthy fat.)

Food sources containing omega-3 include sardines, salmon, herring, sea bass, dark leafy greens, walnuts, hemp seed, flaxseed, flaxseed oil, hemp oil, pumpkin seeds, chia seeds, walnut oil, wheat germ oil, omega-3 fortified eggs, and grass-fed beef.

Another healthy way to obtain omega-3 is supplementing with a high-quality fish or krill oil.

What about Omega-9?

Omega-9 fatty acid is a monounsaturated fat that is also known as oleic acid. It is not considered an "essential" fatty acid because of our body's ability to produce it in small amounts. However, this can only happen if the essential fatty acids (EFAs), omega-3 and omega-6, are present. If the body is low on one of these EFAs it cannot produce enough omega-9. In this instance, omega-9 transforms into an essential fatty acid because of the body's inability to produce it.

While omega-9 is very important, it plays a smaller role than the essential fatty acids omega-3 and omega-6. Primarily, omega-9 has a positive health effect on the lowering of cholesterol levels and, like omega-3, promotes healthy inflammation responses within the body. Other major health benefits of omega-9 are the improvement of immune function and protection against certain types of cancer.

Foods Containing Omega-9

One of the best food sources for omega-9 is olive oil. Other sources include: olives, avocados, almonds, sesame oil, pecans, pistachio nuts, cashews, hazelnuts, and macadamia nuts.

Getting Enough Good Fatty Acids

The body uses short-chain fats to create long-chain fatty acids, which contribute to health in different ways. One of the long-chain fatty acids that the body can make from alpha-linolenic acid is DHA (docosahexaenoic acid), which is critical to brain and eye development. This is why infant formula is fortified with DHA and why pregnant and breastfeeding women are encouraged to have DHA in their diet, either from a food source or a supplement. EPA (eicosapentaenoic acid) is another omega-3 long-chain fatty acid made by the body that's present in breast milk. Like DHA, it's also found in fatty fish.

Several factors affect the body's production of DHA, including the amount of omega-6 fat, saturated fat, and trans fat in the diet. While the body uses omega-3s to create DHA and EPA, there are food sources—mostly fish—that will help make sure you are getting adequate amounts.

Fish that contain the highest amounts of DHA are: salmon, sardines, herring, and rainbow trout.

It's important to note that walnuts and other vegetarian sources of omega-3's such as chia seeds, flaxseeds, and hemp seeds do not provide EPA and DHA. Salmon and other oily fish do not make their own EPA and DHA. No human or animal can make these on their own. The fish acquire them by eating the algae that make EPA and DHA. Your best source of omega-3 is in the form of the fish mentioned above or a fish oil supplement. Andrew Weil, MD, recommends that everyone can benefit from two to four grams of a good fish or krill oil supplement each day.

Healthy Cooking Oils

Healthy cooking oils that are least damaged by high temperatures are sesame oil, coconut oil, ghee, and yes…butter. Also, try cooking lower and slower (200° F) to preserve the oil's many health benefits. It's best to not fry food at all. Steaming is healthier than frying. A word of caution regarding canola oil: it has to be partially hydrogenated or refined before it is used commercially and consequently is a source of trans fats.

Trans Fats: The Silent Killer

Trans fats have skyrocketed in Western diets. In 2006, the FDA required labeling of trans fats on all food packaging. Trans fats are often called "hydrogenated" or "partially hydrogenated oil" on a food label. Trans fats are the bad guys. The main products from which we get trans fats are margarine, shortenings, shortening oils, all of which are made from partially hydrogenated vegetable oils.

These fats promote chronic disease and inflammation by interfering with enzymes involved in making the EPA and DHA in omega-3, the natural inflammatory fighters.

Some cities and states have now outlawed the use of trans fats. There is no controversy anymore regarding the health dangers of these artificially saturated fats; a diet high in hydrogenated fats contributes to chronic inflammation.

Hydrogenation manipulates vegetable and seed oils by adding hydrogen atoms while heating the oil, producing a rancid, thickened oil that extends the shelf life of processed food.

The refining process gives potato chips their crispiness and baked goods their softness. Even a small amount of these fats induces a chemical reaction that may be harmful to your health.

These "bad" fats increase the risk for certain diseases while "good" fats lower the risk. Many times this is not necessarily related to the type of oil used, but rather the quality of the specific product. For example, supermarket corn oil is usually oil that has been heated to a high temperature and chemically treated with various compounds.

On the other hand "unrefined" organic corn oil that has been extracted without chemicals, and has not been heated, refined, or filtered can be beneficial.

In the United States, fast-food french fries typically contain about 40% trans-fatty acids and many popular cookies and crackers range from 30% to 50% trans fat. Doughnuts have about 35% to 40% trans-fatty acids.

These completely unnatural man-made fats cause dysfunction and chaos in your body on a cellular level. Studies have linked trans fats to:

- Cancer: They interfere with enzymes your body uses to fight cancer.
- Diabetes: They interfere with the insulin receptors in your cell membranes.
- Decreased immune function: They reduce your immune response.
- Problems with reproduction: They interfere with enzymes needed to produce sex hormones.
- Obesity: Trans fats contribute more to weight gain than other types of fat.
- Heart disease: Trans fats can cause major clogging of your arteries. Among women with underlying coronary heart disease, eating trans fats increased the risk of sudden cardiac arrest threefold.
- Trans fat is also known to increase blood levels of low-density lipoprotein (LDL), or "bad" cholesterol, while lowering levels of high-density lipoprotein (HDL), or "good" cholesterol.
- Trans fats interfere with your body's use of beneficial omega-3 fats, and have been linked to an increase in asthma.

Be sure to look for hydrogenated or partially hydrogenated trans fats hidden in these foods:

- margarine, shortening
- many commercial baked goods (i.e. crackers, cookies, donuts)
- pancake and cake mixes

- frozen waffles
- pizza dough
- non-dairy creamers
- potato chips and microwave popcorns
- ice cream
- chocolate
- candy
- hot cocoa
- taco shells
- baby foods
- fish sticks and other frozen breaded foods
- instant noodles
- flour tortillas
- processed cheeses
- when trans fats are processed: vitamins, minerals, fibers, and essential fatty acids are destroyed.
- aluminum (involved in making trans fats) and fractions of it remain in the final product.

It would be wise to note that the U.S. Food and Drug Administration (FDA) allows food manufacturers to round to zero any ingredient that accounts for less than 0.5 grams per serving. So while a product may claim that it does not contain trans fats, food manufacturers have lobbied to allow the food to contain up to 0.5 grams per serving.

Saturated Fats

Saturated fats come mostly from animal sources like meat and dairy—fatty meats, eggs, butter, and cheese—and some plant oils like palm oil, palm kernel oil, and coconut oil. Benefits of saturated fat found in healthy, grass-fed, free-range meat are:

1. **Improved cardiovascular risk factors.** The addition of saturated fat to the diet reduces the levels of a substance called lipoprotein that correlates strongly with risk for heart disease.

2. **Stronger bones.** Saturated fat is required for calcium to be effectively incorporated into bone.

3. **Improved liver health.** Saturated fat has been shown to protect the liver from alcohol and medications, including acetaminophen and other drugs commonly used for pain and arthritis.

4. **Healthy lungs.** For proper function, the airspaces of the lungs have to be coated with a thin layer of lung surfactant. The fat content of lung surfactant is 100% saturated fatty acids.

5. **Healthy brain.** Your brain is mainly made of fat and cholesterol. Most of the fatty acids in the brain are actually saturated. A diet that skimps on healthy saturated fats robs your brain of the raw materials it needs to function optimally.

6. **Proper nerve signaling.** Certain saturated fats, particularly those found in butter, coconut oil, and palm oil, send signals that influence metabolism, including such critical jobs as the appropriate release of insulin.

7. **Strong immune system.** Saturated fats found in butter and coconut oil play key roles in immune health. Loss of sufficient saturated fatty acids in white blood cells hampers their ability to recognize and destroy foreign invaders, such as viruses, bacteria, and fungi.

The naturally occurring saturated fat in coconut oil has amazing health benefits. Fifty percent of the fat content in coconut oil is a fat rarely found in nature called lauric acid. Your body converts lauric acid into monolaurin, which has anti-viral, anti-bacterial, and anti-protozoa properties. Here are more health benefits of coconut oil:

- Promoting heart health
- Promoting weight loss
- Supporting immune system health
- Supporting a healthy metabolism
- Providing an immediate energy source
- Keeping skin healthy and youthful looking
- Supporting the proper functioning of the thyroid gland

Michael R. Eades, MD, who has been in full-time practice of nutritional and metabolic medicine, and Joseph Mercola, MD, an osteopathic physician and surgeon, have treated tens of thousands of patients since 1986. Contrary to vegetarian studies, both doctors observed the same results in their practices, that "large numbers of sick people failed to improve when they implemented vegetarian or vegan diets."

Good Fats, Bad Fats Tips

1. Consume mostly omega-3 foods in the form of oily fish, dark leafy greens, walnuts, flaxseed, raw pumpkin seeds, chia seeds, and grass-fed beef.

2. Avoid omega-6 in the form of peanut oil, corn oil, soybean oil, canola oil, margarine, shortening oils, and corn-fed beef.

3. Enjoy healthy omega-9 fats from avocados, olives, olive oil, and nuts such as pecans, cashews, and macadamia nuts.

4. Avoid trans fats (hydrogenated oils); studies show that these contribute to inflammation and chronic disease.

5. Strive for a healthy balance by choosing fats rich in omega-3 and -9 and limiting omega-6.

6. Eat saturated fat from healthy sources such as coconut oil, organic, free range eggs, grass-fed meat, and poultry free of hormones and antibiotics.

7. Eating healthy fats as part of your meal slows down absorption so that you can go longer without feeling hungry.

Fat Facts

1. A fat-free diet, low in protein and high in carbohydrates, elevates insulin levels and promotes fat accumulation since insulin is a fat storage hormone.

2. Essential Fatty Acids (EFAs) are types of fat that are essential in the diet because they cannot be produced by the body.

3. EFAs are vital for healthy brain function, vision, cell communication, and immune system function.

4. Omega-3 fatty acids are the building blocks for 100 billion neurons and a first-line supplement for preventing and reversing inflammation.

5. It is estimated that Americans consume over twenty-five times the level of omega-6 fats as compared to the beneficial omega-3 fatty acids. This imbalance creates inflammation.

6. Omega-6 fats come from a variety of vegetable oils, such as corn oil, but have an inflammatory effect when heated at high temperatures.

7. Hydrogenated fats (better known as trans fats) hide in margarine, commercial baked goods, frozen foods, processed cheese, and candies, and contribute to inflammation and chronic disease.

8. Trans fats start as unsaturated fats and are artificially manipulated into unhealthy saturated fats.

9. Omega-9 has a positive health benefit of lowering cholesterol levels, improving immune function, and protecting against certain types of cancer.

Most Americans get an excess of omega-6 (from processed vegetable oils, snack foods containing such oils, and grain-fed beef) and are deficient in omega-3 (from flaxseed, oily fish, walnuts, dark leafy greens, walnuts, hemp seed oil, hemp seeds, chia seeds, and grass-fed beef). Omega-9 is important but is not considered an essential fatty acid because your body makes it. One of your best sources of omega-9 is olive oil.

Saturated fat in coconut oil and palm oil contain many healthy benefits such as promoting heart health, supporting a healthy immune system and metabolism, and keeping your skin healthy and youthful looking.

In Conclusion

To be healthy, you need to eat fat. The right kind of fat reduces inflammation, supports heart health, healthy immune function, keeps skin and hair healthy, and is critical for brain and eye health. Healthy fats help burn fat.

CHAPTER 25
HEART DISEASE

With a healthy heart, the beat goes on.

Heart disease remains the leading cause of death in the United States. Regardless of the current stage of your health, you can make major improvements by changing your diet and lifestyle to one that promotes health and longevity. In this chapter, we'll explore the contributing factors.

First, let's take a closer look at what causes heart (coronary artery) disease.

Coronary artery disease arises when plaque accumulates in the coronary arteries, the major blood vessels that supply your heart with blood, oxygen, and nutrients. Damage or injury to the inner layer of a coronary artery is caused by a multitude of factors. The plaque accumulating in these arteries is made from various substances circulating in your blood, including calcium, fat, cholesterol, cellular waste, and fibrin, a material involved in blood clotting. This condition causes the arteries to narrow and harden which enables the deposition of plaque and puts one at risk for heart disease. In response to plaque build-up, cells in your arterial walls multiply and secrete additional substances that can worsen the state of clogged arteries.

Eventually, diminished blood flow may cause chest pain (angina), shortness of breath, or other coronary artery disease symptoms. A complete blockage can cause a heart attack. Here are the major risk factors.

Heart Disease Risk Factors

1. **Unresolved emotions.** Deep prolonged anger, frustration, or resentment can trigger inflammation linked to heart disease. Identifying, expressing and releasing unresolved emotions is key.

2. **Smoking.** Nicotine constricts your blood vessels, and carbon monoxide can damage their inner lining, making them more susceptible to atherosclerosis. The incidence of heart attacks in women who smoke at least twenty cigarettes a day is six times that of women who've never smoked. For men who smoke, the incidence is triple that of nonsmokers.

3. **High blood pressure.** Uncontrolled high blood pressure can result in hardening and thickening of your arteries, narrowing the channel through which blood can flow.

4. **Diabetes.** Diabetes is associated with an increased risk of coronary artery disease. Both conditions share similar risk factors, such as obesity and high blood pressure.

5. **Obesity.** Excess weight can heighten risk by increasing levels of the inflammatory factor which is produced and secreted by fat tissue and linked to insulin resistance.

6. **Physical inactivity.** Exercise normalizes your glucose, insulin, and leptin levels which is why lack of exercise is important for heart health.

7. **Metabolic Syndrome.** This refers to a cluster of conditions that includes elevated blood pressure, high triglycerides (a fat dangerous at high levels), elevated insulin levels, and excess body fat around the waist. This syndrome increases the risk of coronary artery disease.

Risk factors often occur in clusters and may build on one another, such as obesity leading to diabetes and high blood pressure. When grouped together, certain risk factors put one at an even greater risk of coronary artery disease.

Below is Helen's story. She illustrates how making diet and lifestyle changes can positively affect one's heart, even after a double bypass heart operation.

How I Beat Heart Disease—Helene G.

In November of 1996, I took a walk as I often did and felt some pressure in my chest. I just thought I was getting a cold. I was sixty-three years old.

The pressure would stop when I stopped walking but one day the pressure didn't stop. I was concerned and called the advice nurse who instructed me to go to the emergency room.

They kept me overnight in the hospital and I was unable to do the treadmill test so they performed an angiogram. My arteries were the size of a pencil and had blockages. That same day they did a double bypass operation.

I had stopped smoking just two months before the surgery. I had a real smoking addiction and was thirty to forty pounds overweight.

I knew I needed to change my diet and my eating habits. I'd heard of Dr. Dean Ornish and I looked him up. He seemed to be the authority on diet and health at that time. His theory was about avoiding fats but he didn't distinguish between good and bad fats then.

I began eating a lot of greens, nuts, and seeds. I would grind seeds into my smoothies. I bought organic food. I had meat a couple times a week such as turkey burgers and occasionally lamb.

I read Dr. Mark Fuhrman's book and increased the nutrient-dense foods that I ate. I had salad every day and cooked greens, seeds, and some meat. I tried to eat five to seven vegetables a day and three fruits a day. I think the nutrient dense diet helped me stay strong. I also ate some yogurt as it helped me feel grounded. I have not had any problems since I made these changes.

Even though I had smoked for forty years and there was heart disease in my family, the lifestyle changes made a big difference. I haven't had any problems or pressure with my heart or chest. I no longer need to get heart tests. My internist doesn't see any problems. My weight is normal now. I try to walk three to four times a week.

I really want to let people know how important it is to eat well and that it is possible to make changes and improve your health at any age. ◆

Emotions and the Heart

There are several theories why a positive attitude is protective for your heart, including that happier people may take better care of themselves and are more likely to lead healthier lifestyles overall.

According to heart surgeon, Mehmet Oz, MD, unresolved emotional and spiritual issues such as anger or a lack of fulfillment can physically affect the heart.

Holistic physician Dr. C. Norman Shealy, states "the most prevalent ongoing emotion leading up heart disease and high blood pressure is chronic anger." These findings parallel those of Stanford University scientists Dr. Bruce Lipton, whose research shows that chronic stress is a primary cause of more than 95 percent of all types of disease conditions. The bottom line of all this research is that effectively preventing and recovering from chronic disease requires healing long-standing unresolved emotional issues.

The connection between optimism and other positive emotions and good health has been firmly established by scientific research, and the link appears to be particularly strong when it comes to heart health. Being "lighthearted," it turns out, is one of the best ways to protect your heart.

Cardiologists at the University of Maryland Medical Center found that laughing can dramatically reduce the risk of a heart attack by curbing unwanted stress. All of your feelings, positive or negative, come with corresponding physiological changes. Your skin, heart rate, digestion, joints, muscle energy levels, the hair on your head, and countless cells and systems you don't even know about change with every emotion. (Stories and ways to release unresolved emotion in chapter 31, Emotions and Health.)

Heart Disease and Genetics

Until recently, it was thought that if heart disease ran in your family, you would be destined to develop heart disease yourself. Recent studies have shown that genetics represent a small fraction of the overall risk factors for heart disease, and all of your risk factors— even the genetic ones—can be altered to help decrease your chances of developing heart disease.

While we share genes and disease such as high blood pressure with our relatives, we often share lifestyles as well. Perhaps your father and his father both had heart attacks. There may be a genetic link, but there is an equal possibility that they shared behavioral risk factors that may not apply to you:

1. Smoking
2. An inactive lifestyle
3. Poor diet

By avoiding these risk factors in your own life, you may be able to play a proactive role in avoiding heart disease.

Gene Activity Changes According to Perception

Our belief system plays a key role. If we think we'll develop heart disease because our father did, then we'll be more likely to do so. However, if we believe that our health lies in the power of our choices and our thoughts, then we're less likely to be affected by our genes.

Science has discovered that thoughts, diet, lifestyle, and environmental exposures control the behavior and physiology of the cell, turning genes on and off. These discoveries run counter to the established scientific view that life is controlled by the genes. Dr. Bruce Lipton, developmental biologist, is best known for promoting the idea that genes and DNA can be manipulated by a person's beliefs.

According to Dr. Lipton, gene activity can change on a daily basis. "If the perception in your mind is reflected in the chemistry of your body, and if your nervous system reads and interprets the environment and then controls the blood's chemistry, then you can literally change the fate of your cells by altering your thoughts."

Dr. Lipton's research illustrates that by changing your perception, your mind can alter the activity of your genes and create over thirty thousand variations of products from each gene. "Gene programs are contained within the nucleus of the cell, and you can rewrite those genetic programs through changing your blood chemistry." In the simplest terms, this means that we need to change the way we think if we are to heal.

Saturated Fats

Saturated fat has been a controversial theme for at least the last decade, but significant findings took place in March of 2013 that may shift the way people think about consuming meat and dairy. *The American Journal of Clinical Nutrition*, one of the most influential journals in biology and medicine, combined the results of twenty-one studies and found that "saturated fat was not associated with an increased risk" of coronary heart disease, stroke, or coronary vascular disease.

In one study, information was recorded from nearly 348,000 participants, most of whom were healthy at the start of the studies. They were followed for five to twenty-three years and were surveyed about their dietary habits. The study's findings concluded that there was no difference in the risk of heart disease or stroke between people with the lowest and highest intake of saturated fat.

Our bodies need saturated fat to stay healthy. Saturated fats from animal and vegetable sources such as organic eggs, organic meats, yogurt, kefir, butter, coconut oil, and palm oil provide a concentrated source of energy in our diet and provide the building blocks for cell membranes and a variety of hormones and hormone-like substances.

The "Fear of Fat" Era

In recent years, we have heard that avoiding foods like eggs and burgers will protect our hearts. A study named "Seven Countries" was conducted in the 1950s and 1960s by nutrition research pioneer Ancel

Keys. He developed a principle that linked dietary fat to coronary heart disease. We were all led to fear fat, specifically in the form of saturated fat coming from meat and dairy. For decades, Keys' conclusions influenced U.S. dietary guidelines and urged the American public to eat a low-fat diet and cut out butter, red meat, animal fats, eggs, and other so called "artery-clogging" fats from their diets. This was a radical change at that time.

As Americans cut out nutritious animal fats from their diets, they began eating more carbs, processed grains, sugars, and high-fructose corn syrup, all of which are nutritional disasters. This type of diet eventually led to increased inflammation and chronic disease.

The cause of chronic inflammation is due to items such as:
1. Consuming refined sugar and carbohydrates
2. Eating trans fats (hydrogenated or partially hydrogenated oils)
3. A sedentary lifestyle
4. Smoking
5. Sustained high emotional stress that leads to high cortisol levels

The Vegetarian Theory

There are many theories for preventing and reversing heart disease. The Vegetarian Theory is one of the most popular today.

According to the Physicians Committee for Responsible Medicine, The China Study (see the Cancer Chapter Part 1) and various other studies, say that vegetarian and vegan diets lower the risk of heart disease. One study published in *Public Health Nutrition* tracked the dietary habits of 592 African-American participants from the Adventist Health Study-2 and categorized them into three eating patterns: vegetarian/vegan, pesco-vegetarian (allow fish in their diet), and non-vegetarian.

Those who consumed a vegetarian/vegan diet had fewer heart disease risk factors including lower blood pressure, half the risk of diabetes, and a 44% reduced risk for hypertension, compared with those who consumed pesco-vegetarian and non-vegetarian diets. Additionally, vegetarians and vegans were 43% less likely to be obese, compared with non-vegetarians. Other important factors not known in this study are whether this group exercised, cut out junk food, addressed unresolved emotional issues, etc.

This study emphasizes the positive effects plant-based diets may have toward disease prevention.

More Studies

A meta-analysis published in the *American Journal of Clinical Nutrition* (2010) pooled together data from twenty-one unique studies that included almost 350,000 people, about 11,000 of whom developed cardiovascular disease (CVD). These people were tracked for an average of fourteen years, and the studies concluded that there is no relationship between the intake of saturated fat and the incidence of heart disease or stroke.

Dr. Dwight Lundell, a heart surgeon with twenty-five years' experience, has performed over 5,000 open-heart surgeries. Dr. Lundell states, "The injury and inflammation in our blood vessels is caused by the low fat diet recommended for years by mainstream medicine."

According to Dr. Lundell, the biggest culprits of chronic inflammation are the overload of simple, highly processed carbohydrates (sugar, flour, and all the products made from them) and the excess consumption of omega-6 vegetable oils like soybean, corn, and sunflower that are found in many processed foods. These are important points to consider.

To Eat or Not to Eat Meat

To eat or not to eat meat has become a sensitive issue for many people. We make choices to eat certain foods based on philosophical, environmental or personal reasons. There are humanitarian and ecological reasons to avoid a meat-centered diet, especially if the meat comes from factory-farmed animals. While we believe that to be an important part of the decision process, we also believe it is equally important to listen to the feedback that your body provides you when you consume a certain diet.

If your current diet allows you to function at the highest level of energy and you rarely feel hungry or crave sweets and you're in good health, that is sign that you are eating food appropriate for your nutritional type.

Our Philosophy

We advocate a whole foods, plant-based diet that includes some saturated fat (animal protein) *if* it energizes you. Each person must determine for themselves if eating meat is right for them. Most people do well making whole, fresh, organic vegetables and fruit a large part of their diet. (If you have a chronic illness, candida, or are prone to weight gain, eat more vegetables than fruit.)

We hold firm to the belief that the biggest enemies of a healthy heart are high amounts of processed white sugar, high fructose corn syrup, processed carbohydrates, trans fats (hydrogenated), and even polyunsaturated vegetable oils (from soybean and corn oil, for example). Development of heart disease, inflammatory response and all of our "Western" diseases are accelerated by these unhealthy foods.

We each need to find our own comfort zone on the spectrum from vegan to the meat-eating "low-carb" enthusiast (for example, the Paleo diet or the Atkins diet). If you choose to eat meat, select the highest quality organic, grass-fed, free range, humanely raised, cage free product to ensure the meat is free of cruelty, hormones, pesticides, and antibiotics. When it comes to meat, quality matters.

In addition, saturated fats act as carriers for important fat-soluble vitamins A, D, E, and K (see benefits below). Saturated fats are needed for the conversion of carotene to vitamin A, as well as for mineral absorption and a host of other biological processes.

Vitamin Benefits of Saturated Fats

1. **Vitamin A.** Essential for vision. Lycopene may lower prostate cancer risk. Keeps tissues and skin healthy. Plays an important role in bone growth.

2. **Vitamin E.** Acts as an antioxidant, neutralizing unstable molecules that can damage cells. Protects vitamin A and certain lipids from damage. Diets rich in vitamin E may help prevent Alzheimer's disease. Supplements may protect against prostate cancer.

3. **Vitamin D.** Aids in cell–to–cell communication throughout the body. Helps maintain normal blood levels of calcium and phosphorus, which strengthen bones. Helps form teeth and bones. Supplements can reduce spinal fractures.

4. **Vitamin K.** Activates proteins and calcium essential to blood clotting. May help prevent hip fractures.

The myth that vegetable oils (rich in omega-6 fats) are healthier for you than saturated animal fats has been tough to dismantle. Vegetable oils such as peanut oil, soybean oil, and corn oil degrade into oxidation products such as free radicals and degraded triglycerides. While people are beginning to understand the problem with unsaturated vegetable oils, they are not yet embracing that saturated fats are beneficial.

In an analysis in 2010 by the International Agency for Research on Cancer (IARC), part of the World Health Organization (WHO), a total of 130 volatile compounds were isolated from a piece of fried chicken alone. One compound is called an "aldehyde" which interferes with DNA. Another is formaldehyde, which is extremely toxic. Kathleen Warner, an oil chemist, who worked with the USDA for more than three decades and directed the committee on heated oils for years, confirmed that aldehydes are toxic. The solution may be a return to stable, solid animal fats like butter and lard which don't oxidize the way vegetable oils do and don't clog up cell membranes as trans fats do.

Gary Taubes' book, *Good Calories, Bad Calories: Challenging the Conventional Wisdom on Diet, Weight Control and Disease,* has done more than anyone to deconstruct the Ansel Keys myth that linked dietary fat to coronary heart disease (referred to in the Good Fats, Bad Fats chapter).

Taubes' conclusions resonate with our views on fat and sugar:

- Saturated fat is not a cause of obesity, heart disease, or any other chronic disease. The problem is the carbohydrates in the diet, their effect on insulin secretion, and thus the hormonal regulation of homeostasis—the entire harmonic ensemble of the human body. The more refined the carbohydrates, the greater the negative effect on our health, weight and well–being.
- Sugars—sucrose and high-fructose corn syrup specifically—are particularly harmful, probably because the combination of fructose and glucose simultaneously elevates insulin levels while overloading the liver with carbohydrates.
- Through their direct effects on insulin and blood sugar, refined carbohydrates, starches, and sugars are the dietary cause of coronary heart disease and diabetes.
- They are also the most likely dietary causes of cancer, Alzheimer's disease, and other chronic diseases of modern civilization.

There has been increasing evidence that added sugars in foods contribute to heart disease.

According to a study of more than 6,000 adults by Emory University and the Centers for Disease Control and Prevention, published in April 2013 in *The Journal of the American Medical Association,* sugars appear to lower levels of HDL cholesterol (the higher your HDL, the better) and raise triglycerides (the lower the better).

High Cholesterol: An Indicator of Inflammation

In the United States, the idea that cholesterol is bad for you is a "fact" we've all been led to believe. Cholesterol and heart disease have been considered almost synonymous for the last half-century. But this theory stops short of seeing the big picture. When doctors see increased cholesterol circulating in your bloodstream, they conclude that it's the cause of heart attacks, not the underlying damage to your arteries. However, a growing number of doctors believe that this is a harmful myth that needs to be dispelled.

Ron Rosedale, MD, an internationally known expert in nutritional and metabolic medicine, points out that "cholesterol is a vital component of every cell membrane on earth. You cannot make estrogen, testosterone, cortisone, and a host of other vital hormones without cholesterol."

Paul M. Ridker, MD, of Harvard Medical School, found that elevated blood levels of C-reactive protein (a substance that increases in the presence of inflammation in the body) increase the risk of heart disease by 4.5 times, a "relationship far stronger than that between cholesterol and heart disease."

Inflammation has been linked to numerous diseases. Conventional medicine is opening to the idea that chronic inflammation can trigger heart attacks, but it continues to blame cholesterol as being the major culprit for heart disease.

If you have increased levels of cholesterol, it is at least in part because of increased inflammation in your body. The cholesterol is there to do a job: help your body to heal and repair.

Weston A. Price Foundation is a U.S. non-profit organization dedicated to restoring nutrient-dense foods to the American diet through education, research, and activism. Sally Fallon, president, and Mary Enig, PhD, an expert in lipid biochemistry, have gone so far as to call high cholesterol "an invented disease, a 'problem' that emerged when health professionals learned how to measure cholesterol levels in the blood."

Conventional medicine misses the mark when it recommends cholesterol-lowering drugs as the way to reduce your risk of heart attacks. It's important to know there is a risk to your health when using cholesterol-lowering drugs. One needs to address what is causing the body damage leading to increased inflammation and ultimately increased cholesterol.

So the real culprit behind arterial plaque is not cholesterol but inflammation.

Inflammation and Heart Disease

The process of inflammation begins when damage occurs to the lining of our arteries. Chemicals are released, arteries constrict, blood becomes more prone to clot, white blood cells are called to the area to eat damaged debris, and cells adjacent to those damaged cells multiply. Ultimately, scars form and inside our arteries we call it plaque. The constriction of our arteries and the "thickening" of our blood further predisposes us to high blood pressure and heart attacks.

We advise including omega-3 fatty acids in your diet to reduce overall inflammation, and taking a high-quality fish oil or krill oil supplement if you're not eating oily fish as a regular part of your diet.

Health Benefits of Omega-3

- Acts as a natural blood thinner
- Helps improve the body's utilization of insulin
- Lowers blood pressure
- Helps the passage of nutrients into cells
- Assists in the elimination of toxic wastes
- Prevents cardiac arrhythmias

Additional Ways to Lower Inflammation and Heart Disease Symptoms

1. **Reduce grains and eliminate sugars in your daily diet.** It's especially important to eliminate high fructose corn syrup.

2. **Eat the right foods for your nutritional type.** You can learn more about your nutritional type by taking a test (www.mercola.com).

3. **Eat healthy fats** such as: Olives and olive oil; coconut oil for cooking, organic dairy products including butter or ghee (instead of margarine or vegetable oil spreads) and yogurt or kefir (goat dairy is easier to digest); avocados; raw nuts and seed; eggs; and organic, grass-fed meats.

4. **Exercise regularly.** Sedentary people run twice the risk of developing heart disease as active people.

5. **Avoid smoking.** If you are a smoker, try to cut down as soon as possible. The sooner you stop, the better off you will be.

6. **Limit alcohol intake.** For women, limit to one alcoholic beverage per day. For men, limit to two per day.

7. **Reduce stress.** High stress on an ongoing basis leads to higher rates of heart issues. (See final chapter for ways to reduce stress.)

8. **Lose excess weight.** The relationship between excess body weight and heart disease has been proven.

With the above information, you have options for reducing inflammation along with lowering high cholesterol levels and the very welcome "side effects" of increased energy, mood, and mental clarity.

Reduce Heart Disease Risk with the Mediterranean Diet

Research published in *The New England Journal of Medicine* (2013) released a study consisting of more than 1.5 million healthy adults who demonstrated that following a Mediterranean diet was not only helpful in reducing risk of death from heart disease and cancer, but also helped reduced incidence of Parkinson's and Alzheimer's diseases.

What is it about the Mediterranean diet that makes it so healthy? A diet rich in fruits, vegetables, nuts, fish, and healthy oils provides thousands of micronutrients, antioxidants, vitamins, and minerals that can help protect against heart disease as well as cancer and Alzheimer's disease.

The key here is the absence of sugar, refined carbohydrates, polyunsaturated vegetable oils, and trans fats (hydrogenated fat).

Heart disease experts say the research results were a triumph because it showed that diet was powerful in reducing heart disease risk, and it did so using the most rigorous methods. Scientists randomly assigned 7,447 people in Spain who were overweight, smokers, or had diabetes or other risk factors for heart disease, to follow the Mediterranean diet.

Monounsaturated fats, found in avocado, fish, and olive oils, are anti-inflammatory and fight disease at the cellular level. According to a study published in *The New England Journal of Medicine*, it is the positive interaction or synergy between all the foods that leads to health benefits.

Studies have shown that it's never too late to adopt the Mediterranean lifestyle to increase longevity and reduce the risk of chronic disease. Research published in *The Journal of the American Medical Association* found that seniors who led a healthy lifestyle—defined as not smoking, eating a Mediterranean-type diet, drinking alcohol in moderation, and engaging in thirty minutes of daily physical activity—significantly increased their life expectancy.

The good news is that we don't have to move to the Mediterranean to reap the benefits of this diet and lifestyle. You can embrace a heart healthy lifestyle by making similar food choices whenever you live.

Facts

1. Trans fats and polyunsaturated omega-6 fats contribute to heart disease by increasing inflammation.

2. Omega-3 fats reduce heart disease through lowering serum triglyceride levels and decreasing blood-clotting tendencies.

3. New research suggests that as little as 500 mg of krill oil may lower your total cholesterol and triglycerides and will likely increase your HDL (good) cholesterol.

4. **Resveratrol**, an antioxidant in red wine, has shown to be beneficial to the heart, when consumed in moderation.

5. Studies show the **Mediterranean diet** is protective against heart disease and obesity due to its high proportion of plant foods, fish, and olive oil. High in fiber, this diet slows down digestion, reduces insulin resistance, and improves insulin sensitivity.

6. **Positive well-being and disposition** reduce heart attack and coronary events by one-third, according to recent studies. Meditators experience positive genetic changes (such as reduced inflammation) following mindfulness practice.

Dr. Bruce Lipton's research illustrates that by changing your perception, your mind can alter the activity of your genes and create over thirty thousand variations of products from each gene. In the simplest terms, this means that we need to change the way we think if we are to heal.

There are controversial studies on whether or not saturated fat contributes to heart disease. When people make a conscious decision to go on a plant-based diet, they most likely eliminate junk food, refined sugars, trans fats, and unhealthy oils. We believe the elimination of these foods is the key to heart health, not the elimination of saturated fat.

For heart health, an anti-inflammatory diet emphasizes whole foods (think single ingredient foods such as sweet potato, an egg, celery, an avocado).

We recommend high quality protein (both plant and animal protein), healthy fats, and organic fruits and vegetables. This will keep your blood sugar levels relatively stable, which in turn lowers both fat deposition and heart-disease risk. (More on "healthy fats" in the Good Fats, Bad Fats chapter.)

Research continues to demonstrate that being physically active and eating a nutritious diet of primarily whole foods that are filling and satisfying can enable people to control weight, lower blood pressure, and reduce the risk of diabetes and heart disease.

Because coronary artery disease often develops over decades, it can go virtually unnoticed until it produces a heart attack. However, there's plenty you can do to prevent and treat coronary artery disease. Start by committing to a healthy lifestyle.

In Conclusion

Reducing heart disease risk factors is paramount to heart health.

A heart healthy diet consisting of high quality protein (both plant and animal protein), healthy fats, and organic fruits and vegetables will keep your blood sugar levels stable, and lower your risk.

Each of us must find the fuel that is most beneficial for our minds and bodies. Combine your optimal nutrition approach with stress reduction and positive thinking and you have a better chance of looking forward to a healthy heart for many years to come.

CHAPTER 26
IRRITABLE BOWEL SYNDROME AND INFLAMMATORY BOWEL DISEASE

You can *control your IBS, not vice versa.*
—Heather Van Vorous

Irritable Bowel Syndrome (IBS)

Do you experience bloating, excessive gas, lower abdominal pain or discomfort, nausea, or alternating bouts of constipation and/or diarrhea? If so, you're not alone. You may be suffering from Irritable Bowel Syndrome (IBS) or Irritable Bowel Disease (IBD).

IBS is classified as a *functional* gastrointestinal disorder, which means there is some type of disturbance in bowel function. It is not a disease, but rather a syndrome, defined as a group of symptoms. These typically include chronic abdominal pain or discomfort and diarrhea, constipation, or alternating bouts of the two. People with IBS may also have other functional disorders such as fibromyalgia, chronic fatigue syndrome, chronic pelvic pain, and temporomandibular joint (TMJ) disorder.

IBS does not cause inflammation, while IBD does. IBS sufferers show no sign of disease or abnormalities when the colon is examined. IBS does not produce the destructive inflammation found in IBD, so in many respects it is a less serious condition. It doesn't result in permanent harm to the intestines, intestinal bleeding, or the harmful complications often occurring with IBD. IBS affects up to 20% of the population, with a higher prevalence in women. IBS is second only to the common cold as a cause of absenteeism from work. It is estimated that it results in direct and indirect medical costs of over $20 billion annually. Causes are thought be to multi-layered, involving diet, infection, antibiotics, and stress.

Irritable Bowel Syndrome Symptoms

It's important to verify that your symptoms match those of Irritable Bowel Syndrome (IBS) before you accept this diagnosis. As noted above, IBS is characterized by continuous or recurrent lower abdominal pain or cramping (from mild to excruciating) in association with altered bowel motility (diarrhea, constipation, or both). Attacks may strike suddenly at any time of day or night, and occasionally—though not typically—wake you from a sound sleep. Gas and bloating are common, but vomiting is not, though it can occur due to nausea from the pain.

Upper GI symptoms are not a typical part of irritable bowel syndrome and neither are passing blood, running a fever, swollen extremities, and joint pain. These symptoms point to other disorders.

It's important that the following diseases are excluded before you accept a diagnosis of Irritable Bowel Syndrome:

1. Colon or thyroid cancers
2. Inflammatory bowel diseases (Crohn's and ulcerative colitis)
3. Bowel obstructions
4. Diverticulosis/diverticulitis
5. Gallbladder problems
6. Food allergies and intolerances
7. Celiac (a genetic, autoimmune disorder resulting in gluten intolerance)
8. Bacterial infections and SIBO (small intestine bacterial overgrowth)
9. Intestinal parasites
10. Endometriosis
11. Ovarian cancer

Below is a story from Colleen, on how she diagnosed her IBS condition and how diet proved to be her greatest weapon in managing her symptoms.

How Diet Helped My IBS—Colleen H.

About two years ago, I contracted what I thought was either traveler's diarrhea or food poisoning. In order to start the process of elimination, I visited the doctor for an upper and lower GI exam, followed by a bowel movement check-up. No problems could be detected, but I was prescribed several different medications. I have found that doctors often prescribe pills that do not help the underlying problem.

After a discussion with Angie Lambert, we suspected it might be irritable bowel syndrome. Luckily, she gave me all the necessary information to change my diet and control the problem.

Following the plan we came up with, I can now control my diarrhea with the proper foods.

I have come to enjoy new foods, including goat cheese and goat products, as well as dairy substitutes, such as almond or rice milk. My diet focuses on sources of soluble fiber, such as oats, rice, and potatoes. I avoid whole-wheat food items, raw greens, and fatty, greasy foods. From this standpoint, IBS and the changes I've made to my diet are a blessing in disguise. My high blood pressure has lowered considerably, which I contribute to my better diet.

Though the cause of my condition remains a mystery, I have found that following the IBS diet really works. I feel fortunate that my condition isn't painful, as many people experience. When I choose to eat foods that I know will trigger diarrhea (for example, ice cream or a hamburger), my bowels move and rumble rather loudly. This is a clue to take a remedy to avoid a diarrhea episode. So I take over-the-counter diarrhea pills or Pepto- Bismol, liquid or tablets, which provides relief.

I often travel with my own snacks and food, which is very helpful in avoiding a diarrhea episode. I'm grateful that I'm in good health and have the energy and vitality to fly all over the U.S., visiting and enjoying my children and grandchildren. ♦

Irritable Bowel Disease (IBD)

Inflammatory bowel disease (IBD) is a group of inflammatory conditions of the colon and small intestine. The major types of IBD are Crohn's disease (CD) and ulcerative colitis (UC). The main difference between CD and UC is the location and nature of the inflammatory changes. Crohn's can affect any part of the gastrointestinal tract, from mouth to anus. Ulcerative colitis, in contrast, is restricted to the colon and the rectum.

These conditions are covered in greater detail below.

What Is Crohn's Disease?

The disease, named after Dr. Crohn, may go by other names, indicating exactly where in the intestines the diseased portion is located. Sores or lesions appear on the surface of the mucosa, the innermost layer or lining of the intestines. The mucosa absorbs salts, water, and other substances while releasing mucous. The different layers of the bowel wall can become inflamed.

Generally, the symptoms of the disease include abdominal pain that can range from cramps to sharp, localized pains; a change in bowel motility such as diarrhea or constipation; blood in the stool; reduced appetite; fever; and fatigue. Other symptoms may include painful abscesses and resulting fistulas, vomiting, nausea, and weight loss.

There are a number of medical treatments that are effective in reducing or controlling inflammation in Crohn's disease patients. There are surgical options when the medical efforts fail, when abscesses or fistula occur, or scar tissue threatens to block intestinal openings.

Dietary changes can be highly effective. Jordan S. Rubin, author of *The Maker's Diet*, writes about his triumph over Crohn's disease with an emphasis on diet and supplements. Rubin promotes the use of probiotics as "good" bacteria that restores balance to the enteric microflora-bacteria that live in the intestines. Lactobacillus preparations and live-culture yogurt can also be beneficial in increasing friendly bacteria in the intestine.

What Is Ulcerative Colitis?

Like Crohn's disease, ulcerative colitis manifests itself in the mucosa. Changes in the mucosa lead to the inflammation and ulceration that causes a disturbance in the absorption of salt and water. This malabsorption leads to diarrhea. Damage to the mucosa can also lead to excessive amounts of mucous in the fecal matter. The ulcerations cause bleeding, which can lead to anemia. Abdominal pain, fever, fatigue, loss of appetite, and weight loss often accompany the disease as well.

There are a number of medical treatments, which include anti-inflammatory drugs that can be effective in reducing or controlling the inflammation process. There are also surgical options if medical efforts fail, such as when scar tissue blocks intestinal openings. As a last resort, there is a cure for UC that involves removing the colon, rectum, and anus, leaving the patient with a stoma opening in the abdomen.

However, dietary changes need to be explored first as in Sheri's story below. Sheri first experienced symptoms of ulcerative colitis at the age of thirteen. Looking back, she can see how stress played a role in the onset of her symptoms.

Overcoming Ulcerative Colitis—Sheri M.

At the age of thirteen, with the usual stress of teenage years and complex family dynamics, I began having symptoms of ulcerative colitis. My parents took me to a few different doctors, but looking back now I can see that conventional Western medicine was merely treating the symptoms and not the real cause of my inflammatory bowel disease. I was prescribed a variety of pharmaceutical drugs that caused unwanted side effects with minimal improvement.

I had flare-ups on and off through my teenage and young adult years, as well as during both of my pregnancies. I worked with various doctors and eventually went to a gastroenterology specialist at UC Medical Center in San Francisco. When I asked him about diet, he simply said "if something bothers you, don't eat it." I came to realize that even gastroenterologists had minimal training in nutrition. It amazed me that many doctors that work with the digestive system seldom discuss food options with their patients.

I started doing my own research and began learning about the effects of gluten and dairy on my digestive system. I found the Specific Carbohydrate Diet (SCD) by Elaine Gottschall, author of *Breaking the Vicious Cycle*, to be very helpful in reducing my symptoms. I eventually eliminated gluten from my diet by baking muffins and breads with almond flour. These were actually delicious and even my friends considered them a yummy treat.

As I changed my diet, I soon noticed improvement in my symptoms. Changing my diet was challenging at first, but as I began to feel better and see the positive effects, I became motivated to continue my new way of eating.

As time went on, I added other complimentary therapies, which included reducing stress in my life through meditation/guided imagery, gentle yoga, spending time in nature, journaling, etc.

I have been free of UC symptoms for many years. I now have the freedom to enjoy many foods. My diet mostly consists of vegetables and some fruit; quinoa; brown rice; lentils; nuts and seeds; meat and fish; and cultured dairy products such as kefir, yogurt, and small amounts of goat cheese and sheep (feta cheese).

Most importantly, I maintain a diet free of gluten and, except for occasional special treats, free of sugar as well. ♦

Nutritional Therapy

There are many effective ways of controlling and reducing IBS and IBD symptoms through diet. Although Western medicine often recommends pharmaceutical drugs, dietary changes are a safe and effective way to manage both IBS and IBD.

Paying special attention to what you eat goes a long way in reducing IBS/IBD symptoms and promoting healing in the gut. It also plays a role in the underlying inflammatory process.

Understanding Soluble vs. Insoluble Fiber

One of the most troublesome pieces of advice routinely given to people with IBS is "eat more fiber." It prompts the question, "What kind of fiber?"

Most people are never even told that there are actually two types of fiber. The term "fiber" in general refers to a wide variety of substances found in plants. Some of these substances can be dissolved in water (soluble fiber) while others do not dissolve (insoluble fiber).

Insoluble fiber is a powerful GI tract stimulant. Although this has the crucial benefit of reducing the colon's exposure to carcinogens, it can also trigger severe attacks of pain and diarrhea in IBS sufferers.

Once you are aware of the general dietary IBS/IBD guidelines, it will be easier to pinpoint which foods cause digestive problems. Here is an abbreviated list of foods that one can safely eat (soluble fiber), foods to eat with caution (insoluble fiber) and foods that will likely trigger an IBS/IBD symptom. This chart is a good starting point to determine if symptoms can be reduced with diet.

Types of fiber to eat and foods you want to avoid with IBS or IBD.

Safe	Caution	Avoid
rice	whole wheat	red meat
pasta	whole grains	dairy
oatmeal	seeds	egg yolks
white breads	nuts	fried foods
rice cereal	popcorn	dark poultry
corn cereal	eggplant	oils
quinoa	beans	shortening
potatoes	lentils	fats
beets	citrus	coffee
squash	dates	chocolate
mushrooms	bell peppers	caffeine
avocados	peas	alcohol
bananas	lettuces	artificial sweeteners
mangoes	onions	fizzy beverages
papayas	garlic	
	leeks	
	shallots	

Eliminating certain trigger foods may be all you need to do to successfully manage your symptoms. The only way to see if any of these recommendations has value for you is to give it a try.

Keeping a food and symptom diary over several weeks will aid you in understanding the foods you are able to tolerate and not tolerate during the time of a flare-up. This helps you see if there are any patterns in your diet that are causing symptoms.

We've covered IBS and IBD; now let's look at another inflammatory bowel condition that is thought to overlap with IBD.

Diverticular Disease

Two bowel-related conditions, diverticulosis and diverticulitis, fall into their own category outside of IBS and IBD. However, there is now thought to be an overlap between chronic diverticular inflammation and IBD.

Diverticulosis and diverticulitis are also called diverticular disease. Diverticular disease is when people have small pouches in their colons that bulge outward through weak spots, like an inner tube that pokes through weak places in a tire. The condition of having diverticula is called diverticulosis. It's estimated that about half of all Americans age sixty to eighty have diverticulosis. When these pouches become infected or inflamed, the condition is called diverticulitis. This happens in 10 to 25% of people with diverticulosis.

IBS and diverticular disease can cause similar symptoms, but they arise from different pathologies. While the medical treatments for the two disorders are different, dietary strategies for minimizing pain are the same.

Soluble fiber, on the other hand, soothes and regulates the digestive tract and is the single greatest dietary aid for preventing IBS symptoms.

If you are suffering from an IBS condition, we recommend the book *Help for IBS* by Heather Van Vorous or her website www.helpforibs.com to learn how symptoms can be minimized with diet.

Heather suggests an organic acacia soluble fiber product which gives IBS and IBD sufferers relief and in many cases more freedom to eat insoluble fiber foods. In addition, you will find an "IBS Cheat Sheet" listing soluble foods, insoluble foods and the foods to avoid. This cheat sheet can be emailed directly to you for free by logging on to www.helpforibs.com and requesting it.

IBS, IBD, and Stress

Although the symptoms of IBS and IBD can most easily be addressed with diet, stress also triggers or exacerbates attacks. Stress inhibits the sympathetic nerve plexuses (aids in the control of most of the body's internal organs) while stimulating excessive adrenaline production, which upsets the rhythmic muscle contractions of the gastrointestinal tract.

Facts

1. Approximately 20% of the population has an IBS condition.

2. Insoluble fiber is a very powerful GI tract stimulant and can trigger severe attacks of pain and diarrhea in IBS/IBD sufferers.

3. Soluble fiber soothes and regulates the digestive tract and is the single greatest dietary aid for preventing IBS/IBD symptoms.

4. There are a number of medical treatments that are effective in reducing or controlling inflammation in Crohn's disease patients.

5. The use of probiotics (good bacteria) can restore balance to the enteric microflora-bacteria that live in the intestines.

6. The two most common IBD conditions are ulcerative colitis and Crohn's disease. Both are serious inflammatory conditions that can be better managed with diet.

7. Approximately half of all Americans age sixty to eighty have diverticulosis.

Tips to Minimize IBS/IBD Symptoms

1. Make soluble fiber the basis of all your meals and snacks when having a flare-up.

2. As symptoms decrease, try insoluble fiber in small portions and never on an empty stomach.

3. Keep a food and symptom diary over several weeks to determine the foods you are able to tolerate and not tolerate (trigger foods) during the time of a flare-up.

4. Avoid trigger foods as much as possible.

5. Join an online IBS/IBD community to ask questions and get answers.

6. Drink fennel tea and peppermint tea. They are both tummy soothers.

7. Practice stress reduction techniques such as yoga or meditation.

In Conclusion

IBS and IBD encompass a variety of conditions of the bowels. IBS does not involve inflammation while IBD does, making IBD a more serious condition.

IBS cannot usually be self-diagnosed, as there are many other disorders that mimic IBS symptoms. Most doctors prescribe medication without making dietary recommendations for relief of symptoms. As shown in Colleen and Sheri's stories, following an IBS/IBD-friendly diet can help one better manage these conditions, oftentimes without medication.

Stress reduction techniques can help reduce symptoms and are a wise practice for overall good health.

CHAPTER 27
LEAKY GUT SYNDROME

In order to be healthy, you must have a healthy gut.
—Amy Myers, MD

Leaky gut syndrome (LGS) is a serious health condition involving inflammation of the gut. LGS is not widely recognized or diagnosed by the medical community. Healing leaky gut was a critical part of the healing process for both of us. Multiple food sensitivities are one of the biggest warning signs of leaky gut syndrome.

A Cause of Leaky Gut

Nonsteroidal anti-inflammatory drugs (NSAID) often leads to Leaky Gut Syndrome. Often people take NSAIDs such as aspirin and ibuprofen to relieve discomfort. An excessive use of NSAIDs may result in a shortage of important enzymes that are involved in digestion. This can trigger a downward spiral of allergies or intolerances, igniting inflammation in areas that are weak or genetically vulnerable to tissue damage such as the joints. Len Saputo, MD, has stated that "one Advil can lead to leaky gut for a day."

Pain Meds and Leaky Gut—Angie L.

I took so much (prescription) Motrin and ibuprofen in my twenties for arthritis that I developed leaky gut syndrome. As a result, I developed multiple food sensitivities. I worked with a naturopath who determined that my gut lining was "very porous" and recommended Reuteri probiotic to restore and re-pad the lining of my gut. Within six weeks of taking this supplement along with having a very clean diet, my gut lining returned to a healthy, normal state and I was more tolerant of the foods I had become very sensitive to.

My Experience with Leaky Gut—Sheri M.

A few years ago, I had intense muscular pain in my neck and shoulders. As a result, I took pain medicine (one a day for five days). Soon after, I began having sensitivities to many of the foods I ate. This manifested in itching on my scalp and all over my body. I suspected that I developed a leaky gut as a result of taking the pain meds. So I began a regime of Reuteri probiotic, known for healing a leaky gut, one a day on an empty stomach and within one to two weeks the itching gradually subsided. ◆

How Leaky Gut Begins

Holistic doctors and alternative health care professionals have long recognized leaky gut as a serious medical condition that involves inflammation of the gut. In a state of leaky gut the intestines become more porous. This permits incompletely digested proteins to enter the bloodstream, where they can trigger inflammatory immune reactions and create toxicity in the blood. Once the immune system has tagged such molecules as an offending agent, the immune system will continually be activated each time the substance is introduced to the body. As the immune system "attacks" each substance an immune complex is formed. An immune complex is essentially a component of the immune system bound to the offending substance. This complex increases the thickness of the blood, impairing circulation to some degree throughout the body. As the circulation is impaired, various systems decrease in function, muscles ache, and energy and vitality are decreased.

As time goes on and this problem remains unchecked, the immune system becomes more and more responsive (and confused) to everything including airborne substances and food chemicals (autoimmunity). This situation typically accounts for multiple chemical sensitivity, fibromyalgia, and chronic fatigue syndrome. Allergy-like food sensitivities caused by a leaky gut can worsen pollen allergies and has been shown to increase symptoms of rheumatoid arthritis. The most common irritants to the intestinal tract are an unhealthy diet, medications, stress, alcohol consumption, antibiotics, and heavy metal toxicity. Your body is assailed by chemicals and heavy metals on a daily basis. The most common are mercury, aluminum, cadmium, arsenic, lead, and nickel. These toxic metals can cause or contribute to a long list of diseases.

Microorganisms in the gut are essential for normal function, and these "good guys" are referred to as probiotics. It is said that there are more microorganisms within the gut than there are cells in the human body! In a healthy body, the microorganisms work harmoniously with the body to aid in immune and digestive function and control the overgrowth of pathogenic forms of microorganisms. Consuming an overabundance of simple carbohydrates such as sugar, white flour, and alcohol (alcohol is converted into sugar) feeds forms of yeast.

When Yeast Becomes A Problem

Yeast is always present within the gut, but it can become overfed and overgrown, irritating the intestinal wall with its toxic waste and "root" structures that dig into the intestines. As the yeast becomes overgrown the intestinal immune system becomes more and more weakened. This allows various pathogenic bacteria, fungi, viruses, and parasites to make themselves at home in your gut resulting in what is called dysbiosis. As the dysbiosis (more bad guys than good guys) becomes more and more pronounced and the pathogenic byproducts further degrade your intestinal wall, the pathogens themselves enter into circulation and find a home wherever the immune system is weakest, and the body is most toxic. This is where viruses and other microbes become more and more pronounced and further weaken the body. This makes the person dealing with the problem hypersensitive and his/her body becomes weaker and weaker.

The Solution

Overcoming the problem requires diet modification and probiotics to allow for normal healing. From personal experience, we know that a leaky gut can heal within weeks with proper diet and a high-quality probiotic such as Reuteri (can be purchased online or at a health food store.)

The path back to gut balance begins with the anti-inflammatory diet (see Arthritis chapter) in addition to the following tips.

Tips for Healing a Leaky Gut

- Eat a healthy diet and eliminate sugar and junk food so your gut lining can heal.
- Take a high quality probiotic supplement.
- If you have to take pain medication or an antibiotic, we recommend taking a probiotic as well, but take them an hour apart from each other.

Include these in your diet:

- **Bone broth.** This is soup made with meat (chicken, beef, or lamb) on the bone which makes a broth containing collagen and the amino acids proline and glycine that can help heal your damaged cell walls.
- **Cultured dairy** contains probiotics that can help heal the gut. Unsweetened goat kefir is one option.
- **Fermented vegetables** contain organic acids that balance intestinal pH and probiotics to support the gut. Sauerkraut, kimchi, and kombucha are excellent sources.
- **Coconut products** are especially good for your gut. Coconut oil is easier to digest than other fats so it is better for leaky gut. Also, coconut kefir contains probiotics that support your digestive system.
- **Omega-3** fats such as grass-fed beef, lamb, and wild caught fish like salmon are beneficial.
- **Filtered water** should be consumed throughout the day.

What to Avoid While Healing a Leaky Gut

- Gluten-containing grains, conventional (nonorganic) meat, conventional dairy, and GMO foods
- Unfiltered tap water, pesticides, NSAIDS, and antibiotics—Consult with your physician if these were prescribed for you.
- Simple or refined carbohydrates that spike blood sugar levels rapidly such as sugar, white bread, white-flour pasta, cookies, cakes, crackers, processed snacks like potato chips and sugary soft drinks
- Artificial non-nutritive sweeteners such as aspartame and Splenda—Choose a natural sweetener like Stevia or Xylitol instead.
- Alcoholic beverages since they hinder the functioning of the immune and digestive systems and retard the healing process
- Coffee/caffeine overconsumption can disrupt the body's systems, causing insomnia and digestive irregularity (constipation or diarrhea)
- Monosodium glutamate (MSG) found in many foods as a flavor enhancer
- Hydrogenated or partially hydrogenated oils (trans fats) found in many processed foods, deep-fried foods, fast food, and junk food—Focus on good fats like olive oil, flax oil, coconut oil, nuts, and seeds.
- Foods that contain artificial flavors and colors

Gluten and casein from dairy are very small proteins that will find their way into the blood stream quite easily because of their molecular size. They create immune responses quite readily until the gut is fully healed. Sugar and simple carbohydrates will feed the "bad" guys and weaken your immunity. Because our food has become so adulterated by processing, chemicals, additives, preservatives, and pesticides, more and more people are finding themselves sensitive to various foods, namely gluten, dairy, and sugar.

Facts about Leaky Gut Syndrome

1. In a state of leaky gut, the intestines become more porous which permits incompletely digested proteins to enter the bloodstream where they can trigger inflammatory immune reactions and create toxicity in the blood.

2. Holistic doctors and alternative health care professionals have long recognized leaky gut as a serious medical condition and can provide guidance and may suggest supplements.

3. Leaky gut can account for multiple chemical sensitivity, fibromyalgia, and chronic fatigue syndrome.

4. Allergy-like food sensitivities caused by a leaky gut can make pollen allergies worse and has been shown to increase symptoms of rheumatoid arthritis.

5. Healing leaky gut requires diet modification and probiotics to allow for normal healing.

In Conclusion

Leaky gut is a state when the intestines become more porous. This permits incompletely digested proteins to enter the bloodstream, where they can trigger inflammatory immune reactions and create toxicity in the blood. The path back to gut balance begins with an anti-inflammatory diet (see Arthritis chapter), a quality probiotic in addition to the suggested tips.

CHAPTER 28
OBESITY AND ACHIEVING
YOUR IDEAL WEIGHT

I can and I will.

Have you felt frustrated with trying to maintain your ideal weight? Are you confused about which direction to take? Are you willing to make a quantum leap toward feeling lighter and healthier? If you answered yes to any of these questions, this chapter may give you some new ideas to implement along with stories to inspire you.

Millions of people are fighting the battle of the bulge. Obesity has become a national health crisis in the U.S. Overall, three out of four American adults and one in three children and teens are currently obese or overweight. Obesity is a leading cause of preventable death in the U.S. Extra weight can indeed take a major toll on health; it increases the risks of type 2 diabetes, heart disease, stroke, many types of cancer, sleep apnea, and other debilitating and chronic illnesses.

Overweight and obesity ranges are determined by using weight and height to calculate a number called the "body mass index" (BMI). BMI is used because, for most people, it correlates with their amount of body fat.

- An adult who has a BMI between 25 and 29.9 is considered overweight.
- An adult who has a BMI of 30 or higher is considered obese.

The main culprit is a nation addicted to overly processed foods, sugar, high fructose corn syrup, trans fats, certain vegetable oils, and sugar-sweetened beverages that destroy rather than sustain good health. The dietary recommendations often employed in the U.S. are not working.

Over the years, various diets have led people in the wrong direction. As stated in the "Good Fats Bad Fats" chapter, a fat-free diet that's high in processed carbohydrates keeps insulin levels elevated, which promotes fat accumulation, since insulin is a fat-storage hormone.

It's interesting to note that individuals who have gastric bypass surgery have rapid weight loss, and the radical change in diet almost immediately reduces high blood pressure, high blood sugar, high cholesterol, inflammation, and clotting. We're not advocating surgery for weight loss, but this shows diet alone creates radical changes in the body.

Dr. Robert H. Lustig is an Endocrinologist at the University of California, San Francisco (UCSF) and is a Professor of Clinical Pediatrics. He practices in the field of neuroendocrinology with an emphasis on the regulation of energy balance by the central nervous system and specializes in childhood obesity. He's become well known for his lecture and YouTube video called "Sugar: The Bitter Truth" and his book *Fat Chance*.

Dr. Lustig believes that the obesity epidemic was born out of a "well-meaning yet tragically flawed" belief that fat should be reduced in our diet. This meant altering recipes and adding high amounts of salt and various forms of sugar to enhance flavor. The food industry had to find new ways to make food taste good, and increased the carbohydrate content, specifically sugar.

He also states that our current sugar consumption has increased fivefold compared to a hundred years ago, and has more than doubled in the past thirty years. The reality is that 20-25% of the calories consumed in the United States come from some variation of sugar, which greatly contributes to inflammation in the body. Perhaps this is why some nutrition experts predict our current generation will not outlive their parents.

While achieving one's ideal weight is important, what's more important is the quality of food you put in your body. Dr. Mark Hyman, author of *The Blood Sugar Solution,* states: "Food is information that changes your metabolism and genes. Shifting to a nutrient rich diet that's high in vegetables, fruits, nuts, seeds, beans, and whole grains improves the expression of hundreds of genes that control insulin function and obesity."

Food Sensitivities and Weight

Most people are not aware that several of the common foods they eat every day can be an inhibiting factor in losing weight. As mentioned in the Food Sensitivities chapter, the top food sensitivities are: wheat (gluten), dairy, corn, soy, and sugar.

Many people suffer from what is termed an "addictive/allergic response," which is when a person craves the foods they are sensitive to and eat these foods in order to temporarily feel better.

Sensitivity to a food may not be a full-blown allergy. It is sometimes harder to detect because symptoms are more subtle, while still possibly having a negative effect on the body. Negative effects can include (but are not limited to) weight gain, gas and bloating, fatigue, brain fog, constipation, fluid retention, arthritis, and headaches. Many people who give up gluten, for example, start losing weight immediately.

Avoid Gluten to Achieve Your Ideal Weight

Gluten, like sugar, often hides in processed foods like ready-made soups, soy sauce, candies, cold cuts, and various low- and no-fat products, as well as refined grain products like bread, pizza crust, pasta, cookies, and pastries. Many of these foods are refined carbohydrates, which are linked to weight gain and obesity.

Switching to a gluten-free diet could help you lose weight, particularly if you've been eating a lot of refined gluten-containing foods. When eating gluten-free, be careful that you're replacing these foods with healthy choices, like vegetables and other whole foods.

If you opt for gluten-free foods, like the wide assortment of gluten-free cookies, pasta, and breads that are now commercially available, there's a good chance that you will not lose weight; gluten-free products may still be high in carbs and/or sugar. Being gluten-free does not necessarily make the food healthy or automatically good for weight loss. The key here is moderation.

To determine if you have a gluten sensitivity, eliminate it for a period of four weeks and notice the difference. From our personal experience and coaching, we have seen that many people benefit from eliminating gluten.

Below are two stories that show how giving up gluten and sugar contributed to weight loss. In the first story, Julie lost thirty-two pounds and thirty-eight inches in six weeks by cutting out sugar, dairy, and gluten.

How I Lost Weight by Cutting Out Gluten, Dairy, and Sugar—Julie J.

In the spring of 2013, I decided there had be an easier way to feel better without exercising, cutting out the foods I loved, or breaking all my bad habits (including drinking coffee, being a part workaholic, getting by on little sleep, and having a drink when I felt like it). I was tired of feeling guilty indulging during some of my most fun and memorable moments!

I'm a professional woman and have been very happily married for thirty-eight years to my second husband. We have owned two businesses—a beach bar/restaurant and a coffee bar/cafe. I have always been very active. I have had no major health issues except hypothyroidism for twenty-five years and I started to gain weight in my late fifties and it seemed with the extra weight came some pain in my joints and swelling in my body as well as a decrease in my energy levels. When I hit my mid-sixties, I felt like the happy, fun, positive, caring side of me was losing my energy.

I thought my holistic chiropractor could check out my overall bone health so I went to see her. She knew my weight gain and painful joints were bothering me and recommended a new program that cuts out sugar, dairy, and gluten from your diet.

So I gave up refined white sugar and replaced it with Xylitol (I didn't like the taste of Stevia, though I did try it). I only had a headache the first three or four days and never after that!

The amount of weight you want to lose determines the length of the program. I was in it for approximately six weeks, and in the first week I was amazed by not only how much weight and bloating I dropped, but also by the disappearance of the headaches I used to have when sleeping and awakening. I also had more energy. The best result, however, was that I no longer suffered from any stiffness or joint pain! I was running up and down steps and felt not ten but twenty years younger. I also noticed improved digestion and better and longer sleep patterns.

After trying many diets and pills to lose weight over the years, this one really worked. Some programs offered effective weight loss, but I would still have other health concerns, or the weight would come right back. The combination of eliminating sugar and gluten from my diet probably had the biggest effect on my success.

In total, I lost thirty-two pounds and thirty-eight inches in those six weeks. My chiropractor said that she had many clients in two years doing this similar diet and I broke the record. She said, "You got the results because you were the one who stuck with the program."

Who knew certain foods could cause so many symptoms! I'm grateful to be able to share this story. ◆

Changing My Diet to Low Carb, No Sugar—Sabine B.

At forty-six, I realized that my weight was the heaviest it had ever been, at 191 lb. I knew that I had to change my life and the way I was eating.

For many years, I thought that I was eating all the right things. Lots of vegetables and salads—but also a lot of sugar and carbohydrates. I had pasta, potatoes, and rice dishes every night and ate a lot of bread. In the afternoon, I would eat a pastry or cookie with my cup of coffee.

I finally realized that I had to cut out all the carbohydrates and sugar from my life. I started in October of 2013 and lost twenty pounds in three months, then ten more pounds within eight months.

I substituted sugar with erythritol and made my own desserts and cakes. I completely changed my ways of cooking and eating. For breakfast, I eat low carb bread that I make with almond flour with butter on top, or I buy sprouted breads lower in carbs and jam sweetened with Xylitol, made by Nature Hollow. I also have Greek yogurt with berries.

However, I no longer eat pasta or potatoes for dinner. I have a lot of fun trying new recipes and experimenting with different salad dressings: olive oil and rice, and apple cider vinegar. I also try new vegetables, sometimes eat eggplant/parmesan eggs, cheese, and occasionally tofu.

For snacks I eat nuts and seeds or homemade granola. For lunch, I eat a variety of veggies and avocado. I was a vegetarian for fifteen years, but I occasionally have meat since my body was craving protein in that form.

I feel better and hope to get off my blood pressure medicine soon. I know that this needs to be a lifestyle—and not just a diet—if I want to keep the weight off and feel good and healthy. ◆

Food Addiction

If you crave certain foods like cereals, bread, pasta/grains, and sugar, you may actually be addicted to them, according to James Braly, MD, medical director of York Nutritional Laboratories and author of *Food Allergy Relief.* "People with food cravings may actually have neurochemical and hormonal imbalances that trigger these cravings," Braly says. Food cravings are not a sign of weakness. In fact, the "feel good" chemical, serotonin, can actually contribute to addiction for many people.

"People with a food addiction may have symptoms like headaches, insomnia, irritability, mood changes, and depression,"

Braly says. They can relieve these symptoms—but only temporarily—by eating the foods they crave.

Most often, the foods we crave are sugars and processed carbohydrates. Emotional eaters often crave specific comfort foods like ice cream, pizza, and chocolate. Certain foods (often carbs and sugar) change the brain's chemistry, increasing the level of serotonin. The person gets a temporary feeling of well-being as the blood sugar rises. The pancreas engages to bring the blood sugar level down. If the blood sugar falls too low, this can result in the person feeling tired, light headed, or irritable, creating the craving again which can be a vicious cycle.

Below is a list of common habits that can help you identify whether or not you may be suffering from food addiction.

1. **Emotional Eating.** On occasion, people eat to satisfy an emotional need when they are worried, stressed, anxious, or depressed. Frequent overeating often leads to feelings of guilt. As a result, the anxiety about their overeating causes them to continue to eat even more. This type of emotional eating can quickly become a vicious downward spiral.

2. **Weight Loss & Weight Gain.** Food addicts suffer from poor body image and constantly feel the need to lose weight. Additionally, emotional eaters can go on binges, which makes weight fluctuation increase. They may also diet often, and experiment with new ways to lose weight.

3. **Substance Abuse.** Emotional eaters and food addicts frequently abuse dangerous substances such as diet pills, laxatives, diuretics, and amphetamines, and engage in harmful activities including self-induced vomiting, frequent fasting, and excessive exercise.

4. **Food Obsession.** Being obsessed with thoughts of food or constantly thinking about the amount of food you eat each day and having anxiety regarding food may be signs of food obsession.

If you identify with any of these items, consider talking to a health professional that specializes in eating disorders, or joining an organization such as Overeaters Anonymous or Emotions Anonymous. Also, perhaps looking at ways to raise your serotonin levels in non-food ways will be beneficial to you.

Tips for Raising Serotonin Naturally

To increase your serotonin levels naturally, and help you with weight loss without resorting to a piece of chocolate cake or cookies, try these suggestions:

- Eliminate suspected food allergens such as gluten (wheat, rye, oats, etc.) and dairy products. (See Food Sensitivities chapter for complete listing.)
- Avoid alcohol.
- Avoid stimulants like caffeinated drinks and cigarettes.
- Increase your exposure to natural light or sunlight to one to two hours a day.
- Get thirty to forty-five minutes of exercise daily.

Make sure you get seven to eight hours of deep sleep every night.

Detoxification for Weight Loss

When you emphasize good quality food, exercise regularly, and avoid toxins, your body does a good job of cleansing and purifying itself. Juicing fruits and vegetables can give your digestive system a rest and your immune system a boost, but keep in mind an overly toxic body may go into detox from juicing and can cause side effects such as light headedness, headaches, and fatigue.

If you're set on trying a juice fast, drink only juice from fresh, organically grown fruits and vegetables. Drink at least four eight to twelve-ounce glasses of juice plus plenty of pure water (at least four eight-ounce glasses per day) and, if you like, unsweetened herbal tea. If you're not preparing the juice yourself, buy natural juices without added sugar. The average length of time for a juice fast is –three to five days.

Portion Control

Large portions also play a central role in the current obesity epidemic. A recent series of studies showed how easily people fall into the habit of consuming oversized portions. In one clinical trial, researchers from Penn State University tracked the food consumption of nearly two dozen adults for eleven days.

First, they gave their volunteers standard sized servings. Then they gave them portions that were 50% larger. The participants consistently ate more when they were provided with more to eat. The only limit the participants in this study placed on themselves was for vegetables —they didn't eat as many of them as they did of the other types of food available. Other studies have shown that providing older children and adults with larger food portions can lead to significant increases in food intake. Portions at restaurants are often too big, so split meals with friends or take half the meal home. Discipline around portion control is key to maintaining one's ideal weight.

Metabolic Rate

Metabolism is the rate at which we convert food into energy, in the form of calories, and burn it as fuel in our cells. Energy cannot be destroyed and food is energy so the energy of your food is either used or stored. Your body may quickly convert calories to energy, or it may do it slowly, storing the extra calories. Portion control then becomes important, based on your metabolic rate. As we get older, most of us follow the norm of a gradually slowing metabolic rate with increasing tendency toward storing extra fat.

The only food group you don't have to worry about over-consuming is vegetables, as long as they aren't drenched in oil or butter. Remember, half of your plate should be vegetables. The good news is we can influence our metabolic rate. The best way to speed it up and keep it from slowing down is exercise!

Exercise

Regular exercise will make you feel good both physically and mentally and helps you lose weight. Developing this healthy living habit takes time and effort and in the beginning it may be challenging. It's common to think you don't have time for exercise. But stick to your routine during the early stage. Once you decide it's a priority in your life, you will make time for it.

Regular exercise helps to reach and maintain a healthy weight. If you take in more calories than needed in a day, exercise offsets a caloric overload and controls body weight. It speeds the rate of energy use, resulting in increased metabolism. When metabolism is increased through exercise, you will maintain the faster rate throughout the day.

If you need reasons to get motivated, here is a list of scientifically proven health benefits that regular exercise brings.

- Works as a powerful antidepressant
- Promotes cardiovascular health
- Prevents and controls diabetes
- Lowers blood pressure
- Reduces risk of stroke
- Builds and maintains muscle strength
- Strengthens bones
- Improves sleep
- Improves sexual function

A common pitfall is to forgo exercise on days when you feel tired and lethargic because you think you do not have enough energy for it. A secret, known to those who have become habitual exercisers is that effort creates energy. Don't wait for energy to come when you are tired; create it by expending effort (unless you are dealing with a specific health challenge that requires rest). You can easily prove to yourself that this principle works. Just give it a try!

For cardiovascular fitness, we recommend starting by walking regularly. At first, aim for at least thirty minutes three times a week and work up to forty-five minutes every day. Once you feel that you're in shape, you can consider whether to continue with your walking program or try jogging.

The number of calories burned during exercise depends on the speed at which you jog or walk and whether or not you tackle inclines. Jogging has the potential to use more calories, although the higher impact of jogging places greater stress on the joints than walking. If your body can handle the impact, jogging is fine.

We recommend variety in your workouts. The more you vary the intensity, duration, and even type of exercise (walking, jogging, bicycling, swimming, hiking, dancing), the more physically challenging each workout, the more your muscles are utilized, and the more calories you will burn.

When starting out, and if your budget permits, it's best to work with a trainer who can suggest the exercises that will benefit you the most and teach you how do to them safely. Staying in shape throughout weight training is also a good way to maintain a more vigorous metabolism and keep off those extra pounds. Once you're in the routine of regular exercise, be sure to add stretching, muscle toning, and strengthening to your routine.

In time, days without exercise will not feel quite right or complete, and you'll then know that you've created a solid, healthy, lifelong habit.

Facts

1. Three out of four American adults and nearly one in three children and teens are currently obese or overweight.

2. Obesity increases the risks of type 2 diabetes, heart disease, stroke, many types of cancer, sleep apnea, and other debilitating and chronic illnesses.

3. A nutrient-rich diet that's high in vegetables, fruits, nuts, seeds, beans, and whole grains improves the expression of hundreds of genes that control insulin function and obesity.

4. Most people are not aware that many common foods they eat every day can be an inhibiting factor in losing weight.

5. If you crave certain foods like cereals, bread, pasta/grains, and sugar, you may actually be addicted to them due to the "feel good" chemical, serotonin.

6. Regular exercise helps to reach and maintain a healthy weight and speeds the rate of energy use, resulting in increased metabolism.

Achieving one's ideal weight is easier for individuals who have a specific and compelling purpose, goal, or intention.

People lose weight when they are able to give up eating refined, starchy carbohydrates, gluten, and refined sugars, and focus their diet on organic fruits and vegetables and healthy fats as seen in Gloria, Julie, and Sabine's weight-loss stories.

The other vital component for achieving your ideal weight is regular exercise. It will make you feel good both physically and mentally and there are a multitude of scientifically proven reasons to get moving. Any activity that boosts your heart rate for twenty to thirty minutes or more increases your metabolic rate.

In Conclusion

The reason Americans turn to fad diets is that they want to lose weight while eating their favorite foods.

Transitioning may be hard at first but once you start eating differently and healthier, you will lose your taste for greasy foods, refined carbs, and junk foods. Over time you will enjoy all the other wonderful benefits like increased energy, clearer thinking, smoother skin, and achieving your ideal weight.

When you emphasize good quality food, exercise regularly, and avoid toxins, your body does a good job of cleansing and purifying itself.

CHAPTER 29
TOXINS IN OUR
HOME AND ENVIRONMENT

Love yourself enough to live a healthy lifestyle.

Many of us try to live better lives by eating organic food, drinking filtered water, exercising, and avoiding prescription drugs when possible. We salute those efforts! But it's also very important to be aware of all the toxic chemicals we are exposed to on a daily basis. The average American is exposed to hundreds of toxic chemicals every day, including right in our own homes.

Thanks to modern chemistry, clothes don't cling, underarms stay fresh, food doesn't stick to the pan, hair stays in place, and the list goes on. But such conveniences can come at a price.

When we repeatedly expose ourselves to chemicals, toxins build up in our bodies and sometimes stay there for years. This chemical "body burden" swirls around inside all of us. In just twenty-six seconds after any exposure to chemicals, they can be found in the organs of our bodies.

There are some ways to protect yourself and your families from exposure to these toxins, which will be covered later in this chapter. For now, let's take a look at chemicals and where they are found. Some of these hidden contaminants you may have never heard of, and many cleaning products don't list the ingredients.

Many of these ingredients are cause for concern because they contain carcinogens, known or suspected reproductive toxins, and endocrine disrupters. The endocrine system influences almost every cell, organ, and function of our bodies. It also plays a role in regulating mood, tissue function, metabolism, and sexual function, reproductive processes, and growth and development.

Harmful Ingredients in Household Cleaning Products

1. **Ammonia** can cause irritation to eyes and mucous membranes. It can also cause breathing difficulty, wheezing, chest pains, pulmonary edema (swelling), and skin burns. High exposure can lead to blindness, lung damage or heart attack.

2. **2-butoxyethanol/ ethylene glycol butyl ether** is a solvent in carpet cleaners and specialty cleaners and can be inhaled or absorbed through the skin and may cause blood disorders, as well as liver and kidney damage.

3. **Ethoxylated nonyl phenols (NPEs)** are known as "gender-benders" and are highly toxic to aquatic organisms, for example.

4. **Methylene chloride** is listed as a possible human carcinogen by the International Agency for Research on Cancer and is commonly found in paint strippers.

5. **Naphthalene and paradichlorobenzene** is used in mothballs and moth crystals. These chemicals are listed by California's Office of Environmental Health Hazards Assessment as substances "known to the state to cause cancer."

6. **Silica** is made from finely ground quartz and is carcinogenic as a fine dust. Found in some abrasive cleansers, which are often used on a regular basis around the home from detergents to dental whitening.

7. **Toluene** is used as a solvent in numerous products, including paints, and is listed by California's Office of Environmental Health Hazard Assessment as a reproductive toxin that may cause harm to the developing fetus. Pregnant women should avoid products containing toluene.

8. **Trisodium nitrilotriacetate (NTA)** is used as a builder in laundry detergents. NTA is listed as a possible human carcinogen by the International Agency for Research on Cancer.

9. **Xylene** is found in graffiti and scuff removers, spray paints, and some adhesives. A suspected reproductive toxin that has shown reproductive harm in laboratory experiments, it is also a neurotoxin that can cause memory loss on repeated exposure.

10. **Bleach (sodium hypochlorite)** mixed with acids (typically found in toilet bowl cleaners) reacts with them to form chlorine gas. When it is mixed with ammonia, it can create chloramine gas, another toxic substance. Bleach is capable of irritating the eyes, skin, and respiratory tract often by simply inhaling the gases it emits. This inhalation has been noted to deteriorate the lungs and esophagus lining in addition to the scarring of the respiratory tract.

11. **Phosphates** used in dishwasher detergents contain 30-40% phosphates. Some also contain high levels of chlorine-based sanitizing ingredients. Phosphates decrease the oxygen that is needed for healthy aquatic life, and contribute to the pollution of bodies of water.

12. **Hydrochloric acid or trichloroethane or lye** are ingredients in drain cleaners. Lye is caustic and burns skin and eyes. If ingested, it will damage the esophagus and stomach. Hydrochloric acid is corrosive and is an eye and skin irritant; it also damages the kidneys, the liver, and the digestive tract. Trichloroethane is an eye and skin irritant and nervous system depressant.

13. **Petroleum distillates** are used in furniture polish, are highly flammable, and can cause skin and lung cancer.

14. **Phenol** is found in furniture polish and air fresheners. When it touches the skin it can cause it to swell, burn, peel, and break out in hives. Even a small amount can cause cold sweats, convulsions, circulatory collapse, and coma.

15. **Nitrobenzene** can easily be absorbed through the skin and is extremely toxic. This chemical can cause skin discoloration, shallow breathing, vomiting, and death. Repeated exposure can cause genetic changes, birth defects, cancer, liver, kidney, heart, and central nervous system damage.

16. **Formaldehyde** is found in air fresheners and mold and mildew cleaners. It is highly toxic and a known carcinogen. It is also an irritant to eyes, nose, throat, and skin. It may cause nausea, headaches, nosebleeds, dizziness, memory loss, and shortness of breath.

17. **Sodium hypochlorite** is a corrosive, irritates or burns skin and eyes, and causes fluid in the lungs which can lead to coma.

You can begin to see how our bodies have become overloaded with chemicals! There is another way!

Avoiding Toxic Cleaning Products

What can you do to avoid and protect yourself and your family from toxic cleaning products? It is easy to go out and buy the standard products you've been using for years, perhaps out of habit and without thinking about it. But because our bodies are accumulating these toxins on a daily basis, the time has come for us to think about the products we use in our homes.

Cleaning products can be among the most hazardous chemicals in your home or office and are therefore regulated by the Consumer Product Safety Commission. These products create hazardous waste—threatening human health and the natural environment.

Cleaning Tips

1. Use one product at a time. It's safest to buy products where all the ingredients are listed. For example, when chlorine bleach comes into contact with ammonia, it creates a hazardous chlorine gas and death can result from mixing chlorine bleach and ammonia.

2. Look for "green" and non-toxic cleaners that don't contain chlorine, alcohols, triclosan, triclocarban, lye, glycol ethers, or ammonia. Choose ones that say "petroleum-free," "90% biodegradable in 3 days," or "phosphate-free," "VOC-free," and "solvent-free."

3. Use hydrogen-peroxide. It is a bleaching agent that doesn't actually contain bleach. Use in your laundry instead of chlorine bleach. Hydrogen peroxide kills mold and mildew, sanitizes counters and cutting boards, and removes stains from counters.

4. Use chlorine-free products to eliminate health risks. Several years of long term, low level exposure to chlorine bleach can negatively affect one's organ systems and health.

5. Borax and baking soda are safe alternatives that can clean and disinfect and are much cheaper than name brand cleaners cleaning products.

Non-Toxic Cleaning Products

If you buy products, a growing number of commercial non-toxic home cleaning products are available as healthier and environmentally responsible alternatives. Using these products, in addition to helping you and your family, helps promote the growth of green businesses, which contribute to a sustainable environment and economy.

Making Your Own Alternative Non-Toxic Cleaners

Adding essential oils to your homemade products is optional, but can be a bonus. Essential oils can disinfect, purify, and even remove stains—all without any toxic chemicals in the mix. Essential oils are naturally antimicrobial and antibacterial.

Kitchen Cleaner

What You'll Need

Baking soda with a damp cloth, essential oil (lemon), plastic flip top container

Preparation

Fill a plastic flip top container halfway with baking soda. Add fifteen to twenty drops essential oil (lemon). Stir. Add more baking soda until it reaches the top of the shaker. Secure the lid and shake to mix. Don't use too much or you'll need to keep rinsing and wiping.

Floor Cleaner

What You'll Need

Distilled white vinegar, filtered water, essential oil (peppermint)

Preparation

Fill a squirt bottle with equal amounts vinegar and water. Add fifteen to twenty drops essential oil (peppermint). Mix. This cleaner can be used on finished wood, ceramic tile, and vinyl.

Tub and Tile Cleaner

What You'll Need

1 2/3 cups baking soda, 1/2 cup liquid soap (Dr. Bronner's liquid soap is a chemical-free product.)

1/2 cup water, 2 tablespoons distilled white vinegar

Preparation

Mix baking soda and liquid soap in a bowl. Dilute with water and add vinegar. Mix with a fork until any lumps are gone and mixture has a pourable consistency (you may need to add more water). Pour into a 16-ounce squeeze container (the kind with a squirt flip-top lid). Shake well before using.

Glass Cleaner

What You'll Need

1/4 cup distilled white vinegar, 1/2 cup liquid soap, 2 cups filtered water

Preparation

Mix soap and water in a clean 16-ounce spray bottle. Add vinegar. Shake well. Once you have cleaned your windows a couple times with this formula, omit the soap (which removes the waxy residue left behind by conventional cleaners) and switch to 1/2 cup of vinegar mixed with 2 cups water.

All-Purpose Cleaner

What You'll Need

2 tablespoons distilled white vinegar. 1 tablespoon Borax, 16 ounces Hot water, 1/4 cup liquid soap

Preparation

Mix and use as needed.

Skin Care Products and Cosmetics

Skin care products and cosmetics are another area of concern. In addition to using non-toxic cleaning products, we need to be cognizant of what we're putting on our skin and in our bodies.

Whether or not you have chemical sensitivity, toxins accumulate in your body all the time, including through our skin, our largest organ.

Vicki Saputo, RN and radio show co-host shares her dramatic story of sensitivities to chemicals in a book written by her husband, Len Saputo, MD, titled, *A Return to Healing.* Here is her story.

My Story—Vicki S.

In 1988, I developed hives. This was the beginning of several years of many recurring serious episodes characterized by hives, itchy burning palms, abdominal pain and cramping, diarrhea, nausea, vomiting, burning sensation in the groin, vibrations in my hands, flushed ears, swollen tongue, swollen feet, and Sternal pain. I also experienced fainting, swollen lips, burning and itchy tingling in my feet and the back of my knees and scalp, red and burning eyes, and anxiety characterized by shivering and hyperventilation.

I never knew when I was going to have another attack or how severe it would be. They occurred unpredictably—in the shower, after eating, when I woke up on an empty stomach. They were completely random. I always carried my adrenalin emergency pack, EpiPen, and often had to give myself an injection.

One of my worst attacks occurred in Hong Kong. I almost died. We had dinner at the Shangri–La Hotel. When we arrived at our room and began packing for our trip home the next day, I felt that familiar burning in my eyes and my palms began to itch. As I was telling my husband, Len, who is an MD that I was starting an attack, I broke out in hives, got diarrhea, my tongue started filling up my mouth, and my speech became slurred. I took an antihistamine, but this was before we knew to have adrenalin on hand. I passed out on the bathroom floor. At some point, in my semi-conscious state, I heard him on the phone frantically shouting that he needed adrenalin right away. Apparently the hotel nurse had some, but she said it was only for emergencies. He yelled, "This is an emergency!"

Fortunately, the hotel nurse arrived and gave me the adrenalin injection I needed along with prednisone. My blood pressure rose to

50 systolic and I was able to get into bed. The nurse packed up to leave, but I started having another attack. The second injection did the trick. Early in the morning when I got out of bed, I felt like I was walking on inner tubes because my feet were so swollen.

These anaphylactic attacks were always on my mind whenever I went out because I never knew if, when, or where I would have one. I didn't tell people because I didn't want to scare them. Wherever I went, I would scan the room to decide who I would pick to help me if need be, and where the nearest bathroom was so I could be treated as privately as possible.

I felt that I had no choice but to go along with the recommended medications that could minimize my allergic attacks. I agreed to take prednisone and two antihistamines. A few months later, I fractured both bones in my ankle because of steroid induced osteoporosis. Both of the antihistamines I was prescribed have since been taken off the market because they were found to be associated with an increased incidence of potentially fatal cardiac arrhythmias when taken with erythromycin or fungicides. I began to wonder if the treatment was more dangerous than the disease!

These severe allergic reactions occurred twenty-eight times. My allergist was a sweetheart of a friend who tried everything, including presenting my case at immunology grand rounds at Stanford Medical Center. I had extensive lab testing and scratch tests, but no allergies were discovered. My diagnosis was "idiopathic anaphylaxis." Anaphylaxis (pronounced "a-na-fi-LAX-is") is a potentially severe or life-threatening allergic reaction that can occur very quickly—as fast as within a couple of minutes of exposure to the allergen. Idiopathic anaphylaxis is diagnosed when no specific trigger can be identified after an appropriate evaluation.

Just when a cure seemed hopeless, we were blessed to meet Russell Jaffe, MD, PhD. It was an amazing coincidence that my husband connected with him because one of my husband's patients had a test that he didn't understand. As things turned out, Dr. Jaffe was coming to the Bay area and Len invited him to our home for dinner to discuss his test. After listening to Dr. Jaffe, Len asked if my condition might be better diagnosed with his test. He knew what to do right away! Then I had a special blood test to determine if I had delayed reactions to foods and chemicals.

The test results showed that I was allergic to more than forty-two foods and chemicals that included everything under the sun from garlic to corn to dairy to olive oil, some sugars, pesticides, preservatives, colorings, and ingredients in my skin care products that included my make-up, shampoo, conditioner, toothpaste, lotions, etc. This was the beginning of an extreme regimen that I was not prepared to accept. I couldn't have even a little speck of anything on this extensive list for nine months if I wanted to get over the allergies.

It was comforting that I had a chance of recovery, but also depressing because we had to get rid of almost every food in our kitchen, even my favorites! I also realized I would not be able to eat out and that not only would my diet, personal care products, and cleaning agents be severely restricted, but I would have to take numerous supplements every day, including sixty-four grams of vitamin C.

The next day I began searching for skin care products that were safe for me. That was a major challenge that even continues today. During the process, I realized that a lot of what I ate and put on my skin wasn't healthy anyway and I asked myself, "Why would I want to eat or put these toxins on my skin or in my environment anyway, even if I wasn't allergic to them?" It was then that I promised God that even if I got over my allergies, I would avoid the toxins. My last attack was in 1992 and I have stuck to my promise and have been motivated to educate others about healthy living.

After nine months of strictly adhering to my new diet, skin care routine, cleaning agents, and nutritional supplements, I was over my episodes of anaphylaxis! It was a miracle. Our lives would be changed forever. Not only did my husband and I change our lifestyle, but we began re-assessing how we viewed mainstream medicine and eventually developed a new style of health care called "health medicine" that integrates mainstream medicine with alternative modalities.

Health medicine is an integrative, holistic, person-centered and preventive model that we developed after founding the Health Medicine Forum in 1994. We brought health medicine into clinical practice about a decade ago at the Health Medicine Center in Walnut Creek, CA. Our website, www.doctorsaputo.com, offers integrative health assessments for thirty-three conditions (including allergic conditions such as mine) on our free website, all in audio and video.

We both practice what we preach and have helped other people live healthy lifestyles through our website, Health Medicine Forum, Health Medicine Center, our radio and TV shows, Len's book, *A Return to Healing*, lectures, interviews, and ongoing research.

Living a healthy lifestyle is the most powerful medicine in the universe. So it is critical that we eat healthy, get enough sleep, exercise daily, reduce our stress level, avoid toxic exposures, maintain a healthy weight, and have a meaningful purpose in our lives. The first step to being healthy is to pay attention to the style in which we live our lives!◆

Vicki has compiled a list below of natural and organic cosmetics and skin care products. She reminds us: "Remember your skin is your body's largest organ and more than 60% of what you put on your skin is absorbed into your blood stream. You don't want to absorb hormone disruptors, carcinogens, or neurotoxins. Organic, natural products are recommended with the absence of synthetic preservatives, artificial colors (especially FDCs), chemical fragrances, and chemical additives. Most of the research has been done for you, so go ahead and enjoy these healthy, natural products." She also adds that three common chemicals to especially avoid are phthalates, parabens and petrolatum.

Natural and Organic Cosmetics & Skin Care Products

- Marie Veronique Nadeau—Fresh organic moisturizers, mist, sun screen, etc. www.mariveronique.com. In Berkeley, CA— (844) 633-7093
- 100% Pure—(510) 548-8595, (415) 814-9788, www.100percentpure.com
- Amazon Rain (Lluvia)—(800) 835-0850, www.amazonherbshop.com
- Real Purity—(800) 253-1694 (the foundation and lipstick are my favorites)
- Ann Marie Gianni—(866) 729-9434, www.annmariegianni.com
- Miessence—(415) 793-6412 (Claudia), www.beautyessentials.messence.com
- Benedetta aromatherapy skin care products, (925) 254-1122 or (707) 773-0941
- Annaé—www.annaebeauty.com, (510) 531-5767 (mask, hydrobase, moisturizer with crystals)
- Aubrey—(800) 282-7394 or health food store (powder blush/eye shadow, powder, hair gel, hair spray etc.)
- Dr. Bernd Friedlander (moisturizers, etc.)—(650) 344-9433
- www.YoungLiving.com—(800) 763-9963. Essential Oils, etc. (purification and Idaho Tansy for insect repellents and itching); www.naturesgift.com is another less expensive choice.
- Snow Lotus Aromatherapy—(707) 577-8048 (Essential Oils, "Sinus Clear" works great!)
- Nature's Sunshine—(800) 223-8225 (essential oils and toothpaste)
- Beyond Health—(800) 250-3063 IndiuMagic deodorant, *l'huile de grace* (herbal, floral essential oil combo) www.beyondhealth.com
- Dr. Hauscha—health food stores (mascara, lipcare stick, D.O. Fresh, coverstick, lip liner)

- Yoanna Skin Care Vitamin E combo—(800) 366-4617, www.yoannaskincare.com
- Paul Penders—health food stores (eye liner)
- Hair dyes—Nature Tint, Naturally Beautiful, Color-Me-Naturally, Color Charm and Henna are portrayed to be safe. Beware of para phenylenediamine in hair dyes, especially when combined with hydrogen peroxide. It is in just about all permanent and semi-permanent hair dyes and has been shown to be carcinogenic. Do not use them on eyelashes. Hair dyes have been known to cause blindness. Check the ingredients of all products in the health food store.
- Personal lubricants—(602) 957-7955, SYLK or Benedetta (800) 868-8331, www.moonmaidbotanicals.com, (877) 253-7853 (V.V. Wild Yam Salve)
- Toothpaste (or a toothsoap at www.toothsoap.com)—Weleda in the health food stores. Real Purity, Freelife, Young Living, Nature's Sunshine (websites listed in beginning of list). Avoid sodium lauryl sulfate, fluoride, diethylene glycol, triclosan, and saccharin in your toothpaste.
- Mercola.com for Bug off and sunscreen. See Young Living above—Idaho Pansy/Purification
- Lip Balm—Truebotanica.com
- Love Nectar Potions "Honey Rose Kissing Balm" pleasureheals.net—(800) 369-1365
- Firenze Nail Polish and remover (no dibutylphthalate, tolulene, or formaldehyde). Uses soy and silk. Okay for occasional use. Low toxicity. (888) 345-5788 or (866) 866-1316, www.firoze.com or firoze@firoze.com
- Jayashree for natural cleaning resource guide—(703) 788-5709
- Shower head water purifier—Aqua Flow (800) 873-4321

Websites for Organic Personal Care Products
- http://www.doctorsaputo.com/a/vicki-s-corner
- www.theorganicmakeupcompany.com
- www.safecosmetics.org
- www.thinkbeforeyoupink.org
- www.lilyofcolorado.com
- www.ewg.org/reports/skindeep

In the next section of this chapter, we cover several topics not widely recognized to be harmful to our health: microwave ovens, amalgam dental fillings, and chemical "chem" trails.

Microwave Ovens

There have been numerous reports and inquiries made into the health hazards of microwave ovens. Many people sense it's not a good idea. Words like "radioactive," "nuked," "cancer causing," and "toxic" have been tossed around. Should we be worried or just pass the criticism of the microwave off as another new trend in our "go green" society?

As gratifying as it is to have hot food ready to eat in one, two, or five minutes, let's first take a look at how a microwave oven works.

Microwave ovens work by emitting radio microwaves that affect the cells and molecules where water is present. This causes the cells to move extremely fast and change polarity so that the energy within the cells is transformed into frictional heat, warming or "cooking" food. So why is this dangerous? Molecules or cells in our food are not able to withstand the violent movement that microwaves force them to undergo during the heating process. Our food is weakened and becomes a deformed version of its original self.

Scientific data has been gathered regarding the detrimental effects of microwaves on the nutrients in your food. Studies show that the microwave process converts certain trans-amino acids into a neurotoxin (poisonous to the nervous system) and nephrotoxic (poisonous to the kidneys). Microwaving milk and cereal grains converts some of their amino acids into carcinogens—cancer causing agents directly involved in the increase of cancer cells.

Another study reported a decreased food value of 60-90% of all foods tested and that the human body cannot metabolize the unknown by-products created in microwaved food. Other findings suggest microwaved foods cause stomach and intestinal cancerous growths and are a contributor of the increased rate of colon cancer in the U.S.

A study published in *The Journal of the Science of Food and Agriculture* found that broccoli "zapped" in the microwave with a little water lost up to 97% of its beneficial antioxidants. By comparison, steamed broccoli lost 11% or fewer of its antioxidants. In a study of garlic, as little as sixty seconds of microwave heating was enough to inactivate its allinase, garlic's principle active ingredient against cancer.

A Japanese study by Watanabe showed that just six minutes of microwave heating turned 30-40% of the B12 in milk into an inert (dead) form. This study has been cited by Dr. Andrew Weil as evidence supporting his concerns about the effects of microwaving.

Microwaving can also destroy the essential disease-fighting agents in breast milk that offer protection for your baby. One study showed that microwaved breast milk loses antibodies and that certain amino acids are converted into other biologically inactive substances, fostering the growth of more potentially pathogenic bacteria. Some altered amino acids are poisons to the nervous system and kidneys. More damage was done to the milk by microwaving it than by any other method of heating. Babies are better off waiting a couple minutes for milk to be warmed in a pan on the stove.

We recommend putting your health before your need for quick food. Have a healthy snack to tide you over while you take the time to cook your food the good old-fashioned way. Just because it's common doesn't mean it's good for you.

We have replaced our microwaves with toaster ovens. We find we can still put a meal together quickly. Toaster ovens heat up fast and are quicker to use than a large oven and are more energy efficient, without the harmful effects of emitting radio microwaves. Also, in the summertime when it's hot, a toaster oven will not heat up your kitchen the way a regular oven will.

Amalgam "Mercury" Dental Fillings

Dental amalgam is a pre-Civil War product that some dentists still use in dental fillings.

For more than 150 years, most Americans with tooth cavities have received "silver" fillings to seal the tooth and prevent further decay. But what most patients don't know is that those fillings can contain high levels of mercury and may be causing more problems than they solve.

Mercury is a heavy metal and exposure to mercury can cause a myriad of illnesses, as well as severe damage to the central nervous system and the gut. Most people are surprised to learn that once dental amalgam is placed on a tooth, the mercury off-gases over time and is released in vapor form as the filling ages.

The filling can be in your mouth for decades causing you to inhale tiny quantities of this toxin on a daily basis. It may be necessary to replace amalgam (mercury) dental fillings and remove the heavy metal residue that builds up in the body tissues and organs. Other dental issues that can interfere with your health are toxic root canals and dental cavitations.

In 2008, after years of denying there was anything even resembling an issue of concern regarding dentist practices, the Food and Drug Administration updated their website: "Dental amalgams contain mercury, which may have neurotoxic effects on the nervous systems of developing children and fetuses."

The documentary *Mercury Undercover* discusses the mountain of evidence about mercury contamination, as reported by doctors, scientists, environmental experts, and mercury-poisoned survivors.

So what should we do if we have amalgam fillings or cavities that need repair?

Dental Tips

- First, talk to your dentist about your present fillings and future needs. If he or she doesn't take your concerns seriously, find a biological dentist who will listen and offer you some options.

- Ask your dentist if he uses precautionary measures (that have become standard) in the removal of amalgams containing mercury.

- Existing amalgam fillings can be removed, but experts advise caution. When fillings are drilled out, a very fine amalgam dust is created that makes it easy for large amounts of mercury to be absorbed by the body during the procedure.

- To minimize this risk, make sure your dentist uses a dental dam, irrigation to keep dust down, and maintain a high-speed suction at the site to remove all the dust and filling remnants immediately.

- Seek and use healthier amalgam alternatives when fillings are needed. Many different types of mercury-free, biocompatible options are available.

- To learn more about the issue of mercury in dental fillings, visit Consumers for Dental Choice at www.toxicteeth.org. CDC is a non-profit organization that aims to inform the public about the dangers of mercury amalgam fillings.

What Goes Up, Must Come Down

"Chemtrails" are a controversial topic and one that we feel is worth mentioning. Chemtrails (also known as stratospheric aerosol geoengineering) are chemicals and heavy metals that have been deliberately sprayed at high altitudes directed by the U.S. military. The government admits to chemtrails and claim it's slowing down global warming through spraying them.

The problem with chemtrails is that what goes up, must come down. Chemtrails differ vastly from the usual plane condensation trails (contrails) that evaporate quickly in the sky. Chemtrails do not dissipate quickly.

Aluminum is said to be a major component in these aerosols, along with other toxic chemicals. Pesticide Action Network North America (PANNA) lists aluminum as "toxic to humans, including carcinogenicity, reproductive and developmental toxicity, neurotoxicity, and acute toxicity." Aluminum also has a history of damaging brain function.

If these chemicals are as dangerous as some claim, they may be polluting our waterways and soil while seeping into crops and contaminating livestock, not to mention changing the weather patterns. Plants are especially sensitive to the soil degradation that occurs with chemtrail spraying, creating serious issues concerning our food supply.

If the air we breathe is filled with a dangerous assortment of toxins, then our immune system will be compromised.

Facts

1. Cleaning products can be among the most hazardous chemicals in your home or office. These products create hazardous waste—threatening human health and the natural environment.

2. There are many ways to make your own alternative non-toxic home cleaning products.

3. Studies show a decreased food value of 60-90% of all foods tested and that the human body cannot metabolize the unknown by-products created in microwaved food.

4. "Silver" amalgam fillings can contain high levels of mercury and may be causing more problems than they solve.

5. The Food and Drug Administration now states that, "Dental amalgams contain mercury, which may have neurotoxic effects on the nervous systems of developing children and fetuses."

6. Aluminum is said to be a major component in "chemtrails" along with other toxic chemicals and heavy metals.

7. Plants are especially sensitive to the soil degradation that occurs with chemtrail spraying, creating serious issues concerning our food supply.

In Conclusion

Living in modern society, we are exposed to hundreds of chemicals every day in our food, in the air, and in our drinking water. Chemicals accumulate for years in our body. There are many ways we can reduce our chemical exposure, starting with our choice of household supplies and cosmetics.

We recommend replacing your microwave with a toaster oven, which heats up faster and quicker than a large oven and is a healthier, more energy-efficient cooking option.

Silver "amalgam" fillings can be a health hazard for people who are sensitive to mercury. One can replace their silver fillings with a biological dentist.

CHAPTER 30
ELECTROMAGNETIC RADIATION

Sensitivity to electromagnetic radiation is the
emerging health problem of the 21st century.
—William Rea, MD

There were days not long ago when making a phone call on the road meant stopping at the corner gas station and using the pay phone. We've come a long way since then. Wireless technology has made it almost impossible to escape the continuous exposure to electro pollution.

The age of technology is here to stay, and we are adapting to all the rapid changes. Among these changes is the continuous exposure to electromagnetic radiation (EMR) surrounding us.

Our dependence on the digital world means we're now living in a sea of electrical energy waves, also known as electro-magnetic frequency (EMF) or electro-magnetic radiation (EMR). These energy waves are estimated to be 100 million times stronger than a hundred years ago. The question is, are our bodies ready for this change?

A wave's electromagnetic frequency is directly related to the amount of energy carried by the wave. Low-frequency electromagnetic waves, for example, have small amounts of energy and, therefore, are relatively safe. These are more commonly known as radio waves. Low-frequency waves, such as radio waves and microwaves, have long wavelengths. EMR is energy in the form of transverse magnetic and electric waves or radiation consisting of electromagnetic waves, including radio waves, infrared, visible light, ultraviolet, x-rays, and gamma rays.

Smart phones, Wi-Fi, e-readers, computers, laptops, and powerful cell towers all emit a spectrum of EMR that has consequences. With Wi-Fi, it's almost impossible to escape the "electro smog"—

electromagnetic radiation emitted by all the Wi-Fi, computers and mobile phones.

Before Wi-Fi you could shut off your computer, walk away from it, and no longer be bombarded by the electromagnetic frequencies that computers generate. Now wherever Wi-Fi is present, whether at home, on an airplane, or in a coffee shop, you are being affected twenty-four hours a day.

A growing body of scientific research acknowledges that the greatest threat to our health and well-being is an invisible form of pollution called electro-pollution. Many health issues have been linked to EMR including various cancers (especially brain, eye, ear, and leukemia), miscarriages, birth defects, chronic fatigue, and/or stress, headaches, nausea, heart problems, autism, learning disabilities, and insomnia.

Symptoms of Electromagnetic Hypersensitivity
1. Confusion/poor concentration/memory loss
2. Fatigue and weakness
3. Headache/migraine
4. Chest pain and heart problems
5. Skin itch/rash/flushing/burning, and/or tingling

Below, Kedzi shares her story of how EMRs dramatically affected her health and her life and the steps she took to reduce exposure and improve her health.

My Electromagnetic Radiation Story—Kedzi M.

During the time I lived in the Sedona, Arizona area, I had a busy private practice as an Integrative Functional Medicine practitioner and Biomedical Empath. I was also part of a healing team for people with addictions.

There were virtually no cell towers and electromagnetic radiation was extremely low in the area where I lived during the late nineties through the mid-2000s. My health and energy were great and I had no physical ailments.

Then I moved to a more rural area at the base of a mountain considered to be the center of northern Arizona. The mountain was covered with electric and microwave towers that I didn't realize would end up being a health hazard for me, as they seemed far enough away. My property was surrounded by thousands of acres of land. Still, I was being "rained on" (negatively impacted) by electromagnetic radiation.

After moving into my newly renovated home, I suddenly started having the following symptoms:

- couldn't sleep at night
- couldn't stay awake during the day, due to extreme fatigue
- couldn't walk a straight line
- trouble reading and adding numbers
- developed skin problems
- my psychic abilities were blocked
- body pain that moved around to different parts of my body on a daily basis
- my body was weakening
- blurry vision and brain fog
- experienced confusion and sadness
- menstrual periods abruptly stopped (healthy until moving in)
- used to have a photographic memory but then I couldn't remember numbers, directions etc.
- hormones tanked like a switch was turned off and my hair began to fall out
- when I used my cell phone it felt like an ice pick sensation in my head
- had to reduce my clients to one every four days causing extreme financial stress

Basically, everything had fallen apart in every area of my life.

About a year and a half later, not knowing what to do about these advancing symptoms, a friend came to visit from Canada. I shared with her the trouble I was having and miraculously my visitor told me

I very well could be electro-sensitive. She offered me a Gia Wellness Cell Guard for my phone.

The first thing I noticed immediately was that I no longer experienced the ice pick sensation while using my phone. Instead, it felt like a velvet wave passing through my brain and body. My brain lit up, turned on, as though the main power source to my entire being was once again connected. Within a couple of days, my hormones began functioning again, allowing my menstrual cycle to resume, as though being on hold for a year.

Using the cell guards and wearing the Gia For Life protective pendant helped my cells release toxins that had accumulated in my body. A hair analysis showed toxins were releasing from my body. I decided to move away from this area.

I am now living in Cave Creek, Arizona. I turn off the router and other electronics when I'm not using them to reduce the saturation of EMR. Every six months I replace the cell guard on my phone. I also use protection in my home, car, on my cordless phone, and on my computer. I wear a protection pendant and use an electromagnetic frequency–protected air tube headset with my cell phone.

My health has greatly improved. I am working with clients regularly again, and I am thankful my friend was able to identify the cause of my illness —electromagnetic hypersensitivity (EHS). ♦

(Sheri Miller is a Gia Wellness consultant. If you are interested in learning more about Gia's products, email Sheri at sherijane@gmail.com.)

What Experts Have to Say about EMR

Dr. Robert O. Becker, a medical researcher who specializes in electromagnetic radiation, as well as an author and twice Nobel Prize nominee, is very concerned about electro pollution. In his opinion, the greatest polluting element in the earth's environment at the present time is the proliferation of electromagnetic fields. He considers this to be a health threat on a larger scale than global warming

A study from Sweden suggests that if you started using a cell phone as a teen, you have a five times greater risk of brain cancer than those who started as an adult.

Dr. Thomas Rau, medical director of the world-renowned Paracelsus Clinic in Lustmühle, Switzerland, states, "Of the 10,000 patients our clinic sees annually, 3,000 have electromagnetic hypersensitivity (EHS)." EHS occurs when the amount of EMF radiation exceeds the body's ability to deal with it.

Everyone has an imaginary (but very real) "lifetime radiation cup." The body can only tolerate that amount of electromagnetic radiation. Once that cup is full, because of many small deposits of EMF exposure or even one very large deposit, any exposure can be physically felt and can cause end result illnesses such as fibromyalgia, cancer, MS, chronic fatigue, and more.

According to Dr. Rau, electromagnetic loads can also lead to cancer, ADD, tinnitus, migraines, insomnia, arrhythmia, Parkinson's and even back pain. At Paracelsus Clinic, cancer patients are now routinely educated in electromagnetic field remediation strategies.

Exposing children in schools to radiation, known to impair brain function and learning, Rau describes as "criminal." He says it's unethical to expose children in this way. We know that cell towers, cell sites and Wi-Fi are hurting the brains of children, so to put such stations into schools is "*very, very, very* bad." Rau poses the question: "Does the school, does society, want to have intelligent, well-educated children, or not?"

When patients come to see Dr. Rau complaining of migraine headaches, he first tests for electromagnetic cloud. His team of specialists work together with an instrument that measures the cloud. Then they either identify the outside cloud source or remove problem devices. Portable house phones can cause "electromagnetic clouds." When these are removed, patients get better.

People with heavy metal loads in the body which may come from root canals, amalgam (silver mercury) fillings, or implants tend to suffer more from electromagnetic radiation compared to those who do not. The heavy metals might well be absorbing the EMR.

Bioinitiative Working Group

Numerous scientific studies have been conducted on EMR and brain cancer. The Bioinitiative Working Group released a 650-page report citing more than 2,000 studies that detail the toxic effects of EMFs from all sources. Chronic exposure to even low-level radiation (like that from cell phones) can cause a variety of cancers, impair immunity, and contribute to Alzheimer's disease, dementia, heart disease, and many other ailments. Additionally, every single study of brain tumors that looks at ten or more years of cell phone use shows an increased risk of brain cancer.

Chris Woollams is the Chief Executive of CANCERactive, Britain's top complementary and integrative cancer charity. In an article titled "Cell phones and Brain Tumors—15 Reasons for Concern," he writes, "In a world where a drug cannot be launched without proof that it is safe, where the use of herbs and natural compounds available to all since early Egyptian times are now questioned, their safety subjected to the deepest scrutiny, where a new food cannot be launched without prior approval, the idea that we use cordless phones, and introduce Wi-Fi and mobile phones without restrictions around our five-year-olds is double-standards gone mad. I speak, not just as an editor and scientist that has looked in depth at all the research, but as a father that lost his beloved daughter to a brain tumor."

Paul J. Rosch, MD, and clinical professor of medicine and psychiatry, New York Medical College; Diplomat and on the National Board of Medical Examiners, believes that all communication in the body eventually takes place via subtle electromagnetic signaling between cells. This signaling is disrupted by artificial electro pollution we have not had time to adapt to.

Award-winning scientist and author, Devra Lee states that Professor Joel Moskowitz of University of California Berkeley combined information from all other studies ever done on brain tumors and cell phones. He found "consistent evidence that heavy cell phone use for a decade or longer increases brain tumor risk at least 30%."

More than a dozen countries restrict the use of cell phones by children and advise precautions regarding their use. Nearly all studies of those who have used cell phones for a decade or more have found doubled risks of brain tumors.

Emerging science has discovered that the problem with cell phones does not come from voltage but rather from the information carrying radio wave (ICRW). The body's cells perceive this wave as a dangerous, foreign invader. Instantly, the cell membrane goes into a protective lock down mode, keeping nutrients from being fully absorbed and toxins from getting out. Vital cell-to-cell communication is lost, and the body goes into stress mode.

Specific Absorption Rate

The specific absorption rate (SAR) exposure limit was developed in 1982 in an attempt to set a safety limit that is lower than the level of radiofrequency (RF) exposure known to increase biological response (damage) in animals. These limits were reaffirmed in 1991 and again in 1999. There is a consensus that these limits need to be re-evaluated by the appropriate government agencies.

The current exposure limits that are used by the Federal Communications Commission to set standards were based on that of a military recruit—a 200–pound, 6-foot tall man with an 11-pound head—using a phone for six minutes. The SAR values vary with the source of exposure and size and age of the person using the phone. The limit is 1.6 W/kg, but there are phones on the market emitting higher SAR values. This is why this information should be available at point of sale.

In 2010, San Francisco was the first city in the nation to require warning labels on cell phones. This legislation states that every cell phone retailer must post the level of radiation each phone emits at point of sale with educational materials concerning cell phone radiation also available to the public.

Tips for Reducing EMR Exposure at Work

For many of us, our jobs force us to be in situations where higher than normal EMRs exist. In some situations, EMRs cannot be avoided. Here is how you can reduce your exposure to high EMR levels at work.

1. Text more and use your speaker feature to keep your phone further from your head.

2. Keep your cell phone away from your body when you're not using it. For example, when driving in your car or sitting at your desk, don't have your phone right next to you. Keep it at least three feet away from your body.

3. Keep cell phones out of your pocket and off your body.

4. Don't rest your laptop on your lap since certain cancers such as testicular cancer are on the rise especially among teens.

5. If you are an employer whose employees are exposed to high levels of EMF, you should first and foremost inform all of your employees about the potential dangers of working under such conditions, and ensure them that their safety is your primary concern. Then proceed to take action to lower their exposure.

6. Electromagnetic fields are strongest within three feet of the piece(s) of equipment generating it. Once outside this perimeter, the EMR begins to reduce dramatically.

7. Move your workstation at least three feet away from any EMR source such as electrical panels, equipment banks, and other sources of electromagnetic fields. Try to maintain that distance when working in an environment where there are many pieces of electrical equipment.

8. If you cannot stay entirely clear of EMRs in your daily work, at least try to reduce the amount of your exposure by limiting exposure times.

9. Spread out your office power equipment such as printers, computers, and other peripherals evenly to prevent a buildup of EMR in one area.

10. Turn your phone off when you're not using it or not waiting for an important call. However, for those who rely heavily and sometimes solely on their cell phone for work purposes, protection devices are an option.

11. Protection devices may be attached to your electrical devices to lower EMR exposure both at home and at work.

Tips for Reducing EMR Exposure at Home

There are many steps you can take to reduce EMF exposure for your family inside your home.

1. Turn off your Wi-Fi at night for ten to twelve hours.

2. Cordless phones emit as much or more radiation as our cell phones since they rest on a mini cell tower. If you must use them, use the speaker phone feature.

3. Keep cell phones away from sleeping areas.

Children and Babies

Brain cancer is the number one cancer today among children partially because children's brains are more vulnerable to EMR exposure. Babies are the most vulnerable.

Here are tips for your baby and children.

- Move the nightlight or bedside light well away from the crib/bed.
- Never push extension cables under the bed.
- Don't put a baby or child on a waterbed or electric blanket.

Facts

- Children who began using mobile phones as teenagers have four to five times greater risk of developing malignant brain tumors compared to those who did not use phones at these ages.
- Men who use their cell phones at least four hours per day have been found to have half the sperm count of non-users.
- For the developing fetus, prolonged cell phone use or placing the cell phone on "standby" mode near the fetus significantly increases the risk of learning problems in children and may present other dangers to child development.
- Those who regularly use cell phones with higher radiated power, such as people living in rural areas or using phones in moving cars, face greater risks of brain tumors and other chronic health problems.

- Other serious health problems significantly associated with regular cell phone usage includes: breast, salivary gland, rectal, and testicular cancers, short-term memory loss, sleep and attention disturbances, headaches, hearing loss, cognitive impairments, dementia and even possibly Alzheimer's disease.
- Studies find that cell phone radiation damages DNA, increases abnormal proteins, alters memory, behavior and brain chemistry, and increases the uptake of pollutants into the brain.

Electro pollution is a very real concern to present and future generations. When introduced in the 1980s, cell phones were exempted from pre-market safety testing and were intended for short use by working adults. Over the past decade, millions of children and young people have become regular users. Wireless technology has made it virtually impossible to escape the continuous exposure to electro pollution.

In Conclusion

Electro pollution is a very real concern to present and future generations. When introduced in the 1980s, cell phones were exempted from pre-market safety testing and were intended for short use by working adults. Over the past decade, millions of children and young people have become regular users. The mobile phone industry has not addressed the concerns.

We are not promoting elimination of cell phone usage but we do promote safer usage of all electronic devices to reduce potential long-term chronic health impacts. The best defense is to employ precautionary measures when using devices emitting EMR (as listed above) together with protection devices that can help mitigate the effect of EMR in your home, office and the environment.

We feel it's important to become educated on this important emerging public health issue.

CHAPTER 31
EMOTIONS AND HEALTH

*When it comes to our health, optimistic thoughts may be
more beneficial than all the others.*

Good feelings, scientists now know, have healing effects on the
body and researchers studying everything from the flu to HIV
continue to find eye-opening evidence that a person's mind-set can
influence the immunity and the rate at which one heals from injuries
and illness.

When it comes to our health, there are four basic factors that are
under our control: 1. the quality of our diet, 2. a commitment to
exercise, 3. the quality of our thoughts, and 4. the decision not to
smoke.

Optimistic thoughts may be more beneficial than all the others.
Scientists don't yet fully understand the biological mechanisms at
work, but they know that negative feelings like stress, sadness, and
worry cause a spike in the hormone cortisol, which in turn suppresses
the immune system.

Having a positive outlook and a cheerful disposition isn't only a
happier way to live your life, it's a healthier way as well.

What Is Good Emotional Health?

People who have good emotional health are aware of their
thoughts, feelings, and behaviors. They have learned healthy ways to
cope with the stress and problems that are a normal part of life. They
feel good about themselves and have healthy relationships.

How Can Emotions Affect My Health?

Although it is still often overlooked, emotional health is
absolutely essential to your physical health and healing. When you're

loving yourself and taking good care of yourself, emotional health is easier to experience.

Every time you have a good thought, a happy thought, a hopeful thought, or a kind thought, your brain releases chemicals that make your body feel good and lowers your deep limbic system (DLS). Increase in DLS is associated with depression, dysthymia and negativity. Becoming aware of our thoughts and emotions can increase our understanding of ourselves and of what is involved in being healthy and genuinely happy.

Our emotions have a capacity to harm and heal—not just psychologically but physically. So, just how do feelings affect our health?

Feelings of love help restore the nervous system and improve memory by triggering the growth of new brain cells, according to researchers at the University of Pavia. The feeling of love and contentment induces a calming effect on both the body and the mind. "Love" may be a feeling we associate with another, but love and contentment can also be a feeling we experience within ourselves.

In a study of the effects of laughter, Dr. Lee Berk of Loma Linda University in California discovered that levels of mood-boosting beta-endorphins increased by 27%, while human growth hormone, a substance that aids sleep and cellular repair, rose by 87%. The effects were achieved by watching a humorous film. In another study, the mere anticipation of laughter was enough to reduce levels of the stress hormones cortisol and adrenalin. Norman Cousins, author of several books including *Anatomy of an Illness*, recounts his triumph over a severe illness and the helpful effect that laughing and a positive attitude had on his recovery.

U.S. biochemist Dr. William Frey compared the tears of women who cried for emotional reasons with those whose eyes welled up on exposure to onions. Emotional tears were found to contain high levels of the hormones and neurotransmitters associated with stress. Frey concluded that the purpose of emotional crying is to remove stress chemicals. Holding back tears leaves the body prone to anxiety, including weakened immunity, impaired memory, and poor digestion.

Emotions Play an Important Role in Regaining Our Health

Holistic medical practitioners treat the entire body knowing that psychological and emotional factors and lack of a spiritual connection are as much to blame for the onset of illness as are physical factors.

Everyone carries some form of emotional pain. Most people with a serious illness carry enormous amounts of buried emotional pain, which is then stuffed into the cells and organs of the body. Recent studies in major scientific journals such as the American Medical Association, confirm that holding onto past events and negative emotion can wreak havoc on every aspect of our physical, mental, emotional, and spiritual self.

The good news is that there are numerous ways we can identify and clear our body and mind of counter-productive and emotional issues. Once the mind/body is cleared and thoughts return to positive and joyful feelings, healing is accelerated and chronic pain is relieved. Life again becomes more purposeful, joyful, and fulfilling.

Sheri and Angie each worked to release and clear negative emotions, beliefs, and "programs" as part of their journeys back to health. Identifying negative emotions and characteristics in oneself is critical to recovery. By working through and clearing these emotions each of us was able to regain health more quickly.

Clearing Out Negative Emotion

There are many ways to help clear out stored negative emotion. Our preference is to work with "clearing" therapies, specifically Emotional Freedom Technique (EFT) and Spiritual Response Therapy (SRT) . We found that by working with these therapies, we were able to work through emotions with a greater level of understanding and clear them from the body.

Out of all the different clearing methods we sampled, Sheri most resonated with EFT and Angie with SRT. Two other widely used emotion clearing methods are The Emotion Code (Dr. Bradley Nelson) and Neuro-Emotional Technique (NET).

Neuro-Emotional Technique (NET): A Holistic Approach to Clearing Emotions

Neuro-Emotional Technique (NET) is a holistic approach that combines traditional Chinese medicine, chiropractic, and applied kinesiology that finds and removes unresolved "negative emotional blocks," toxins in the body, and deficiencies in nutrition. Laurie's story below illustrates how clearing an emotional issue can completely clear a physical issue, using NET.

Spontaneous Healing of Fibroids—Laurie D.

I have learned that physical symptoms, which I like to think of as our body talking to us, can be the result of mental, emotional, social, financial, or other stress-related problems. These problems/symptoms can be healed energetically. But what does "healed energetically" mean?

Oftentimes, symptoms can and often do heal spontaneously as a result of earnest prayer or over time, they get better. There is, however, a learned process called spiritual response technique (SRT) as well as another technique called Neuro-Emotional Technique (NET). Both offer a methodical, detailed process to get to the root of a problem using an applied kinesiology (ideometer response) technique to determine the source or root of a symptom/problem. Once identified, the root is removed and the symptom/problem no longer presents itself. This means that the energy causing the symptom is gone so the symptom is also gone.

An example for me was uterine fibroids. My OB-GYN was not able to perform a pap smear due to the size and location of uterine fibroids so he scheduled an ultrasound procedure to recheck them in three weeks' time for eventual surgical removal.

During those three weeks, I visited my chiropractor for nine ten-minute visits with the intention of understanding what was causing the uterine fibroids. Using NET, my chiropractor was able to discern the cause of each fibroid. In my case, this physical symptom was the result of unresolved hurt from prior long-term relationships with my total of four boyfriends. I did not consciously know there was any "hurt or harm" from those relationships. I thought they were fun, enjoyable, happy relationships.

At my OB-GYN three-week follow up appointment, during an ultrasound investigation as to the size and location of the fibroids, the fibroids had completely disappeared. By energetically identifying and clearing emotional issues that settled for me as fibroids in my uterus, I experienced a true and complete physical healing. ♦

(For more information about NET, see www.netmindbody.com.)

How Emotions are Stored in the Body

"Accumulated pain is a negative energy field that occupies your body and mind." —Eckhart Tolle, author of *Power of Now*

At the physical level of every single cell, the body records every experience that is not fully felt or released. The human body is a sophisticated bio-computer. The hardware/body is the anatomy and physiology and the software/belief system is the programming or psychology.

Everyone has a story. We all have hidden memories, resentments, grief, pain, and anger that need to be released from the cells of the body. No one can escape some form of negative experience and most of us don't have the skill set to release the emotions in the moment in which they surface.

What is most interesting about retaining emotion and memory at the cellular memory level is that past-recorded experiences shape our current and future reality. Stored negative emotion recorded into the cells of the body or "cellular memory" influences the way we perform routine tasks and react to stress and emotional challenges in our present situations.

In other words, our buried emotion and sabotaging beliefs and thoughts influence or color our perception of reality. We see through distorted lenses that cause us to react to outside stimulus in sometimes unhealthy or unexplainable ways. We overreact at work with a friend or boyfriend/girlfriend or spouse about something minor, all in response to something that was programmed by another person or situation at another time. In order to see clearly again, we have to clean out these originally programmed moments and their corresponding emotions.

HeartMath and EFT—Sheri M.

I've been a student of HeartMath for several years. HeartMath is a tool that I often use when I'm in a stressful situation.

The core of HeartMath philosophy is that the heart is the key to tapping into an intelligence that can provide us with peace and fulfillment. Science has shown that the heart communicates with the body and brain on various different levels.

HeartMath has taken this information, and translated it into simple tools that focus on teaching us how to listen to, and follow, the intuitive information of the heart. We can learn how to better make decisions, and to use the power of the heart to manage the mind and emotions.

Freeze-Frame is the simplest of the HeartMath tools. It is a one-minute technique that allows a major shift in perception. More than positive thinking, it creates a definitive, heartfelt shift in how we view a situation, an individual or ourselves.

When you're feeling stressed:

1. Shift out of the head, and focus on the area around your heart. Keep your attention there for at least ten seconds. Continue to breathe normally.

2. Recall a positive time or feeling you had in your life, and attempt to re-experience it. Remember, try not simply to visualize it, but rather to feel it fully.

3. Ask a question from the heart: "What can I do in this situation to make it different?" or "What can I do to minimize stress?"

4. Listen to the response of your heart. You may hear nothing, but perhaps feel calmer. You may receive verification of something you already know, or you may experience a complete perspective shift, seeing the crisis in a more balanced way. Although we may not have control over the event, we do have control over our perception of the event.

Learning to achieve and sustain smooth and balanced heart rhythms, what scientists refer to as heart coherence, is one of the healthiest, easiest and fastest ways to improve your quality of life.

I use HeartMath if I'm in a situation where I'm feeling upset about something or in a situation that is challenging. I will focus on my heart by breathing through my heart. Sometimes I'll actually put my hand over my heart. I then recall a positive feeling, often times the love I feel for my grandchildren. This process will shift my energy and assist me in looking at the situation in a more positive way. My emotions feel more balanced and I feel better.

As I healed, I focused on affirmations to regain my health. I stopped describing myself as sick or tired. When I started doing affirmations it felt strange. After a few weeks, I felt like the messages were being embedded into my body, which in fact they were! In time, I truly believed what I was saying. My favorite affirmations included:

- I am happy, healthy, vibrant, and balanced.
- My body is my temple and I honor and love it.
- Money comes to me in expected and unexpected ways.

When you repeat aloud your affirmation or intention, you are recording it into your subconscious mind. Your subconscious mind just does what it's told. It doesn't know any better. Use your subconscious mind to help strengthen your immune system.

Also, whatever I currently desire in my life I create an affirmation around it. For example, I recently manifested the home I wanted as a result of a clear intention and positive affirmation. Thoughts are powerful and we *can* manifest with our thoughts.

I have used EFT at various times to help with physical symptoms or emotional upset. Emotional freedom technique (EFT) is a relatively new discovery and a self-healing treatment within the field of energy psychology. EFT is catching the attention of healers, scientists, spiritualists, and people in general.

EFT is a form of acupressure, based on the same energy meridians used in traditional acupuncture to treat physical and emotional ailments for over five thousand years, but without the invasiveness of needles. Instead, simple tapping with the fingertips is used to input kinetic energy onto specific meridians on the head and chest while you think about your specific problem—whether it is a traumatic event, an addiction, or pain—and voice positive affirmations.

This combination of tapping the energy meridians and voicing positive affirmation works to clear the "short-circuit"— the emotional block—from your body's bioenergy system, thus restoring your mind and body's balance, which is essential for optimal health and the healing of physical disease.

A few times when I had a headache at the end of a stressful day, I used EFT and after a few minutes my headache was greatly reduced or gone. Other times I have used it when I had muscular pain or when I was upset or had a disagreement with someone. It helped me to let go of the pain or the situation and feel calmer and more grounded. ♦

Here's a story of how one mom keeps herself and her two teens well using energy medicine, including Emotional Freedom Technique (EFT).

How EFT Helped My Son—Carol C.

I grew up in the seventies with a mother who studied, researched, and healed using the science of energy medicine. I learned how meridians carried our body's vital energy along intricate invisible pathways located just under the skin. Later I learned how these channels interconnect the physical universe with the pulsing, living tissues inside of us.

The flow of our subtle energy can determine whether we develop illness or not. Along with channels, we also have energetic fields of vibration that link our thoughts and emotions to the physical body, a reminder that what we put into our minds as well as our bodies is essential to whole body wellness.

Understanding subtle energy and the powerful impact it has to support true wellness became my mission, and as an adult, I'm grateful for a life free of prescriptive drugs or malady. My children are also thriving young adults empowered with their own subtle energy tools of self-care. Thanks to my mother who illuminated the way.

The following is an example of how my son was helped by just one simple self-help technique using subtle energy: tapping (the meridians).

Although bright and sociable, my nineteen-year-old son suffered occasional bouts of emotional distress in new social situations. During the high school years we treated this distress with Bach Flower Therapies, and were grateful for the wonderful results.

Several years later, during a college break, he was anxious about seeing old friends from the past. I decided to treat his anxiousness with another subtle energy healing technique, more popularly known as emotional freedom technique (EFT), and now commonly known as "Tapping." This technique is extremely powerful and one of the best self-help methods I know.

A week after this treatment, I received the following text message from my son: "I have to tell you, the 'tapping' thing worked! I've never been more relaxed when I'm in public now. I've just come to the conclusion that I look how I look and that really doesn't matter. And I'm fine with these imperfections because I've kind of come to accept myself. It's weird; it was like this sudden switch."

The beauty of this technique is that in the absence of emotional distress, his light case of acne cleared up. The emotional and physical connection was addressed and healed—without drugs, office visits, or long-term psychoanalysis. ♦

Cycle of Behavior That Stops an Emotion from Happening

Emotional pain in the body is the accumulation of negative emotions and experiences that were not acknowledged or allowed in the moment in which they originally took place. These emotions and experiences were never processed. They were either denied or resisted.

This is a cycle of behavior with the singular effort to resist feeling emotion. We ignore the moment of pain and say, "I will deal with this later. Where's the chocolate, caffeine, wine, or beer?" When emotional pain is stuffed and resisted it can result in the form of physical pain and disease. With willingness and time to determine the right modality, we can release these buried emotions and our self-esteem and physical health will soar.

How Can I Improve My Emotional Health?

Here are nine tips on how to stay positive and healthy.

1. **Express your feelings in appropriate ways.** If feelings of stress, sadness or anxiety are causing physical problems, keeping these feelings inside can make you feel worse. It's okay to let your loved ones know when something is bothering you. However, keep in mind that your family and friends may not be able to help you deal with your feelings appropriately. At these times, ask someone outside the situation—such as your doctor, a therapist, health coach, or a spiritual advisor for advice and support to help you improve your emotional health.

2. **Calm your mind and body.** Relaxation methods, such as meditation, are useful ways to bring your emotions into balance. Meditation can take many forms. For example, you may do it by

sitting, walking, lying down yoga, standing yoga, or simply focusing on your breath.

We know tai chi has all sorts of benefits, and here's one more: In research conducted at UCLA, sixty-one older adults took tai chi classes three times a week, while sixty-one others attended health education classes. At the end of four months, both groups received a dose of the shingles vaccine—and the tai chi group achieved twice the level of immunity. "It's likely to be the meditation component that is causing the effect," says study author Michael R. Irwin, "which means it's possible other forms of meditative exercise, like yoga, would lead to a similar boost."

3. **Lean on your friends.** Sheldon Cohen, PhD, is a psychology professor at Carnegie Mellon University and an expert on the link between social networks and health. In one of his studies, Cohen exposed 276 adults to the common cold virus. He wasn't surprised to find that smokers were three times more likely to get sick. But Cohen also found that subjects who had the least variety of social relationships fared even worse—they were 4.2 times more likely to catch a cold. One reason people with strong social ties are better at warding off infection may be that they have lower stress levels, Cohen says.

4. **Live a balanced life.** Try not to obsess about the problems at work, school, or home that lead to negative feelings. This doesn't mean you have to pretend to be happy when you feel stressed, anxious, or upset. It's important to deal with these negative feelings, but try to focus on the positive things in your life, too. You may want to use a journal to keep track of things that make you feel happy or peaceful. Research has shown that having a positive outlook can improve your quality of life and give your health a boost. You may also need to find ways to let go of some things in your life that make you feel stressed and overwhelmed. Make time for things you enjoy.

5. **Develop resilience.** People with resilience are able to cope with stress in a healthy way. Resilience can be learned and

strengthened with different strategies. These include having social support, keeping a positive view of yourself, accepting change, and keeping things in perspective.

6. **Take care of yourself.** To have good emotional health, it's important to take care of your body by having a regular routine for eating healthy meals, getting enough sleep, and exercising to relieve pent-up tension.

7. **Look on the bright side.** In a recent study, 193 people were assessed to determine their level of positive emotions (including happiness, calmness, and liveliness). Participants were exposed to a virus. The results of the study found that people who scored low on positive emotions were three times as likely to succumb to the bug. What's intriguing about this phenomenon, says Lara M. Stepleman, PhD, an assistant professor of psychiatry and health behavior at the Medical College of Georgia, is that "we all have the ability to choose an optimistic mind-set. And with practice, we can get better at it."

8. **Count your blessings.** Feelings of gratitude boost immunity, lower blood pressure, and speed healing. Dr. Rollin McCraty of the Institute of HeartMath in the U.S. is studying the link between emotions and physical health, and has found that, like love, gratitude and contentment also trigger oxytocin. "Oxytocin is secreted by the heart whenever you feel open and connected," says McCraty. It switches off stress by causing the nervous system to relax. Oxygenation to tissues increases significantly, as does healing. We've found that gratitude is also associated with more harmonious electric activity around both the heart and brain—the very state in which these organs operate most effectively.

9. **Love, bless, and release everyone, including yourself.** Spiritual response therapy (SRT) founder Robert Detzler repeatedly advises, "Love, bless, and release everyone and everything." He elaborates by saying that love is the only true creative energy and that love is the solution to every problem. There is truth in love and falsehood in fear. We don't hurt another by holding them captive

with our resentments or hates, we really only hurt ourselves. Robert states, "Learn to love and bless disease and difficulty so it can dissolve."

If your negative feelings don't go away and are so strong that they keep you from enjoying life, it's important you address it and seek professional help.

On Health and Happiness

Good health and happiness don't come from wealth, perfect looks or even a romantic relationship. Health and happiness come from within. This is why, if we truly want to be healthy and happy, we need to work on ourselves first. Those who are happy and healthy tend to have certain characteristics in common. If we learn to apply these habits in our own lives, there's a good chance we'll be happier, too.

15 Habits of Healthy, Happy People

1. Have self-love
2. Practice forgiveness
3. Treat others with kindness
4. Express gratitude for what they have
5. Speak well of others
6. Don't make excuses
7. Live in the present
8. Maintain a regular sleep schedule
9. Don't compare themselves to others
10. Surround themselves with positive people
11. Take time to listen
12. Nurture social relationships
13. Focus on the positive
14. Practice being honest
15. Eat a healthy diet

40 Ways to Nourish Yourself

Creating a Lifestyle That Feeds Your Spirit

1. **Take a technology break for 30 minutes.** Turn off your phone. Your email, internet, text messages, and voice mail will be there for you when you return to them. The longer tech break, the better.

2. **Go on a media fast.** Many of us feel the day isn't complete until we read the newspaper or check the headline news; yet the news reported is seldom good. Treat yourself to a day without news.

3. **Car meditation.** Pull over in your car on your way home and take at least five minutes to let go of your day and unwind through focusing on your breath.

4. **Retreat to a room and close the door.** Taking a few minutes to be alone can make you feel kinder and happier. Find serenity in the sanctuary of a special room and let your loved ones know you are taking time out for yourself.

5. **Limit television time.** You may find yourself more relaxed without the stimulation of television that can drain energy and add to tension.

6. **Clean out your junk drawer or closet.** Your space affects your well-being. Get rid of things you don't love. Re-creating your space can really free up your energy to allow more flow of joy and abundance.

7. **Do something for someone else.** A single act of kindness strengthens the immune system and raises serotonin in both the giver and receiver of kindness.

8. **Journaling** is a good way to get your thoughts on paper and get in touch with how you're feeling. It can help you identify patterns, statements, or stories you say to yourself.

9. **Massage** can be a great way to ease tension, release toxins and pamper yourself. Foot reflexology can be a less expensive way to go if budget is a concern.

10. **Soak in a warm bath.** Light some candles, put on music or a relaxation CD. Use some essential oils. Relax without guilt.

11. **Create a home altar** as a space to stay in touch with important elements to you…a statue, a rosary, crystals, stones/gems, or a picture or poem that inspires or empowers you.

12. **Walk in nature** (or just walk around the block!) Be it alone, with a friend or an animal companion, fresh air and movement can raise your mood and your energy.

13. **Create a list of intentions/dreams** that make you feel excited when you read them. This process can be very fun and uplifting, especially when you manifest your intention!

14. **Prayer** is scientifically proven to make a difference. It helps you get your mind out of the way and connect with spirit, whatever you perceive that to be.

15. **Dance or sing** at home, in the car, or in the shower. Turn up the stereo, move, and sing out loud.

16. **Exercise classes** are a great way to get and stay motivated, especially participating in group exercise classes such as strength training, boot camp, Nia, Soul Cycle or Zumba.

17. **Teach.** Perhaps there's a subject you're very passionate about. Teaching can be very rewarding and exciting, even if it's on a volunteer basis.

18. **Spend time with a furry friend.** For those of you with pets, you know how nourishing it can be to sit with, pet, and connect with your dog, cat, or other furry friend.

19. **Spiritual groups.** Finding a group to connect with spiritually can be a very fulfilling and joyful experience.

20. **Communing with nature.** Whether at the beach, in the mountains, by a lake, fishing, hiking, or simply sitting on a rock or bench can be a wonderful way to connect with Mother Nature.

21. **Playing with children** can help you connect to your own inner child and remind you to be playful and have fun.

22. **Talking heart-to-heart with a close friend.** Nothing beats talking to a close friend you trust and love. It's good for the soul to be vulnerable, open, and honest, without judgment.

23. **Create a vision board.** Collect things you love, images that inspire, dreams you are creating. Put it where you see it every day. If you saw the movie or read *The Secret*, you know how powerful this can be.

23. **Scrapbooking** can be a fun way to express yourself in a creative activity.

24. **Painting or drawing.** Try taking a painting or drawing class. It's never too late to try something new.

25. **Meditation.** To help you ground, clear your space, relax, and clear your chakras. Buy a CD, take a class, or just sit for five minutes and notice your breath.

26. **Gardening.** Even if you don't have a yard, planting and repotting plants is very relaxing. Gardening is a wonderful way to quiet the mind and connect with the energy of plants.

27. **Affirmations.** Regardless of how you might be feeling say, "I am in perfect health, I am strong today, I feel good today, I am healthy. The healing power of spirit fills every cell of my body." Even if you feel awful, say it anyway. Our subconscious mind can help heal the body.

28. **Take a friend to lunch.** It's fun to treat, and it's also fun to be treated!

29. **Read a good book or listen to an audio book.** Books can inspire you and help you to stay on track and feel positive and optimistic. Whatever your taste, indulge in a good book to nourish your mind and spirit.

30. **Essential oils.** Aromas contained in essential oils derived from botanical sources are used to treat emotions such as stress and anxiety, as well as to enhance health. Oils are great for alleviating pain.

31. **Camping.** Listening to a river flowing right outside your tent, sitting by a fire, gazing at the stars, and listening to the sounds of nature is restful and rejuvenating.

32. **Sailing.** Being out on the water, feeling the wind, and charting your vessel can nourish your spirit.

33. Connect with like-minded people by taking classes to connect, commune, interact, socialize, and create new, nourishing relationships.

34. Learn something new. Taking up something new for the first time in your life such as learning an instrument or a new language can increase self-esteem while building new neurons in the brain.

35. Lighten up and laugh more. You know the old saying "Laughter is the best medicine." If you don't have enough laughter in your life, set the intention to laugh more and you will. Rent a comedy or see a live comedy show.

36. Yoga, which means "union," encompasses a range of spiritual, emotional, energetic, and meditative practices to elicit the relaxation response.

37. Cook a warm, nutritious, delicious meal for yourself and/or your loved ones. Create ambiance by lighting a candle and playing music that's relaxing. Savor and enjoy it. Notice how nourished you feel.

38. Be creative. Write poetry or a song, play the guitar, paint, sculpt, or draw. Use your imagination to unleash your creative side.

39. Gratitude. Practice being grateful and enjoy the good in your life. Gratitude can be a quick way to shift your perspective.

40. Have fun! Activities you enjoy loosen up your energy and bring in optimism. Plan a fun activity or see a funny movie. Life is meant to be joyful.

In Conclusion

Regardless of the method or methods you choose to re-connect with your inner self, know that once you make the connection, life is far more enjoyable.

CHAPTER 32
MEDITATION: A PATH TO WELLNESS

Take this moment.
Relax your shoulders.
Relax your jaw.
Inhale slow.
Exhale slower.
Soften your gaze.
Now be.
Just be.

Meditating is the delicate art of doing nothing and just being—of letting go of everything emotionally and physically. It provides the mind with a much needed, deep rest. Meditation is an act of self-love.

Dr. Wayne Dyer writes in his book, *Secrets for Success and Inner Peace*, that the average person is said to have 60,000 separate thoughts a day. If we could reduce that number even by half, a whole world of possibilities could open up. He states, "Everything that's created comes out of silence. Your thoughts emerge from the nothingness of silence. Your words come out of this void."

The way to cut your thoughts in half or slow them down is through meditation. The mind is known to be a factor in stress and stress-related disorders, and meditation calms the mind and reduces stress. Results are noticeable almost immediately.

Meditation can help us be more mindful of our thoughts which nurtures greater awareness, clarity, and acceptance of the present moment. Mindfulness provides a simple but powerful route for getting ourselves unstuck.

Going to a meditation class is a great way to get started. Whether you download a meditation app or get started with a group class, the most important thing is to begin.

Meditation for Stress Reduction

Mindfulness-based meditation practices have shown beneficial effects on inflammatory disorders and are even endorsed by the American Heart Association as a means of preventative intervention.

Meditation rewires your brain in amazing ways that can positively alter every aspect of your life, from the way you feel about yourself to releasing addiction and depression and reducing pain and inflammation.

Researchers at Massachusetts General Hospital and Harvard University have shown, using MRI brain scanning technology, that eight weeks of mindfulness-based stress reduction (MBSR) leads to thickening of a number of different regions of the brain associated with learning and memory, emotion regulation, the sense of self, and perspective. They also found that the amygdala, a region deep in the brain that is responsible for appraising and reacting to perceived threats was thinner after practicing mindfulness meditation.

Jon Kabat-Zinn, professor of medicine emeritus and creator of the Stress Reduction Clinic and the Center for Mindfulness in Medicine, Health Care, and Society at the University of Massachusetts Medical School states, "When I start the day cultivating some calmness and concentration, I'm more mindful and relaxed the rest of the day and better able to recognize stress and handle it more effectively."

Here is a meditation to help you get started. Notice how little time it takes to evoke the presence of calm and relaxation.

Universal Love Meditation

Sit down and get comfortable. Close your eyes.

Imagine a silver thread from the top of your head up to the ceiling and beyond. Give a gently tug upward on this silver thread to lift and elongate your spine.

Now imagine a grounding cord (a tree, a waterfall or a cylinder of light) connected from the base of your spine to the crystal core of Mother Earth.

State: *I invoke the presence of Universal Love.*

In your mind, imagine a radiant beam of bright light enter your body through the top of your head traveling into your heart.

Feel the warm sensation as the beam surrounds your heart and glows even brighter.

This radiant beam of light is Universal Love coming directly from Source/God.

State: *I merge with this loving, light energy flowing directly from Source/God.*

Keep your focus on the warm feeling of this light energy moving in all directions from your heart.

Follow it through the chest into your neck, head, shoulders and down your arms to your fingertips.

Now allow the warm, light energy to flow down your spine, torso, hips, legs and feet to the tips of your toes.

Invite this loving light to completely envelop you like a warm, soft blanket. ◆

Notice how it feels to make this connection.

Ways to Start Your Meditation Practice

Everyone has experienced a meditative state in certain moments of deep joy or relaxation, perhaps gazing at a sunset or when you are completely engrossed in an activity. Just for a moment the mind becomes calm and at ease. We have such moments and want to repeat them, but don't know how. Practicing a form meditation gives us the ability to recreate this feeling of ease and awareness.

Here are forms of meditation to consider:

1. **Transcendental Meditation.** (TM) is practiced by 5 million people worldwide. TM assists in gaining deep relaxation, eliminating stress, promoting health, increasing creativity and intelligence, and attaining inner happiness and fulfillment. You are given a mantra by a teacher and that mantra is what you use to take yourself deeper while meditating.

2. **Art of Living Meditation** allows the conscious mind to settle deeply into itself. When the mind settles down, it lets go of all tension and stress and centers itself in the present moment. It is only in the present moment that we find true happiness; those moments when we are free from regrets about the past or anxiety about the future. Without effort, our inner nature is available.

3. **Mindfulness Based Stress Reduction (MBSR)** is an eight-week training in mindfulness meditation which cultivates greater awareness of the unity of mind and body, as well as unconscious thoughts, feelings, and behaviors that can undermine emotional, physical, and spiritual health. Practicing mindfulness is a powerful route for getting back in touch with our own wisdom and vitality.

4. **Buddhist Meditation.** This is a very simple practice that has been passed on for 2500 years, from generation to generation. Buddhist meditation encompasses a variety of meditation techniques that aim to develop mindfulness, tranquility, and insight.

5. **Meditation Apps.** Use your mobile phone for meditation apps. Here are a few we like: Omvana, Rest and Relaxation guided meditation, and Calm.

What I Do to Relax—Sheri M.

Over the years, I've meditated in different kinds of ways. I began meditating by listening to guided progressive relaxation CD's that involved tensing and relaxing each of my muscles. As time went on, I was able to elicit this relaxation response on my own without needing to be guided. Eventually, this type of relaxation expanded into more traditional meditation, at first being guided by audio recordings and again eventually being able to meditate on my own.

Currently, depending on my mood, I alternate between listening to meditation CDs or simply focusing on my breath and meditating on my own. If I'm in the car, I park in a shaded area under a tree and meditate. My meditations can last anywhere from five to forty-five minutes.

I've also taken meditation classes and learned how to bring healing energy into my body. Now when I have a few minutes I can quickly get into a state of relaxation by sitting quietly with my eyes closed, sometimes listening to soothing music which can induce relaxation for me. In the morning I do yoga stretches while in a meditative state, and end by surrounding myself with protection and prayer.

At the end of a busy day before going home, I often pull off the road for ten or twenty minutes and listen to a meditation app on my phone called "Rest and Relaxation." Then I'm refreshed, relaxed and ready to enjoy my evening. ◆

CHAPTER 33
ENERGY MEDICINE, ALTERNATIVE MEDICINE, AND MIRACLES

Each healing experience is an adventure in soul growth and
a step toward our eventual destiny.
—Edgar Cayce, Father of Holistic Medicine

In the 1920s, Albert Einstein stated that everything is composed of energy. This reality has been largely ignored by modern society, though things are slowly changing as more scientists are saying the same thing.

We are a bundle of intelligent energy in the form of a human body. We are made up of cells, which are made up of atoms, which are made up of subatomic particles. What are subatomic particles? Energy.

You can heal, restore and revitalize your body and mind with simple energy techniques that are friendly, natural and non-invasive. Energy Medicine communicates with the subtle energy systems of the body, and can repattern the energies at the root of an illness. It offers ways to naturally and systematically reclaim our health and vitality.

Energy medicine involves the invisible forces that animate the human body. Qigong, tai chi, acupuncture, Touch for Health, Reiki, Quantum Touch and hands-on healing are all examples.

Well respected heart surgeon, Dr. Mehmet Oz, spoke to an international audience on Oprah in 2007 and announced that "The next big frontier in medicine is energy medicine."

Society is beginning to reawaken to the forgotten truth that everything is energy and that working with energy is a viable healing option available to all of us. The book *Energy Medicine* by Donna

Eden teaches simple self-healing techniques. According to Donna, the best medicine is energy medicine.

My Miracles with Energy Medicine—Angie L.

It's been very empowering to learn various tools and techniques that help me stay clear and grounded.

My first introduction to "energy medicine" was at a health fair in 2005. I found myself drawn to a massage table where a man was doing free fifteen-minute energy "tune ups." I had experienced sacral pain in my low back since I was a teenager and had seen chiropractors on and off for years. One track season in high school I had to quit due to this low back pain.

When I arrived at the health fair, I was dragging one leg to accommodate the discomfort. I could not sit or sleep in certain positions because it made it worse. So on this particular day I was open-minded without any expectations as I laid down on the massage table while this energy healer ran energy on my back. After my "tune up," I immediately had less pain. So I set up a full one-hour session scheduled for a few days later.

When I arrived at my appointment, the energy healer, Will, warmly greeted me and I lay down on his massage table. He tuned into my low back, specifically my sacrum. He sensed that my sacrum was holding onto a memory of injury due to an accident, not from this life but from a prior lifetime. He cleared the cellular memory of that incident. The pain left my body and never returned. That was thirteen years ago. I can now sit or sleep any way I want without creating pain in my sacrum.

This spontaneous healing opened my eyes and mind to the world of energy, which I now know is everything. Our thoughts are energy, food is energy, trees are energy, and we are energy. Our thoughts can feed us or drain us. They can be high, medium, or low in vibration or frequency. Most of our thoughts are unconscious, but these are the thoughts that run our lives.

I decided I wanted to teach energy healing to people suffering from pain. I met a wonderful woman and master tai chi trainer, Robin, who would become my tai chi instructor and dear friend. I became certified in a sun style form called "Tai Chi for Arthritis" and began teaching at wellness centers, health clubs, and an assisted living facilities.

I also began taking classes at two different intuitive training schools to deepen my understanding of energy, auras, and chakras. Through energy "readings," I learned that I took on other people's junk (negative energy) and processed it through my body. I did not have conscious awareness I was doing this, but this was validated by several energy healers/readers. I continued to deepen my awareness of "energy" and my relationship to energy and others.

Around this time period, I had excruciating pain in both of my legs, making it very difficult to walk. The pain wasn't arthritis, because it wasn't the joints that hurt, but rather the entire leg, both of them. This is after I learned tai chi and was teaching tai chi, meditation, and nutrition classes. I thought to myself, isn't my tai chi practice supposed to be clearing my energy field?

I was tempted to go to a doctor, but instead I called my trusted energy healer, Tom, who helped me understand that I was carrying other people's energy in my legs. As he began to clear their energy out, the pain disappeared. This happened two more times and knowing what it was, I was able to do the clearing myself. The leg pain stopped completely but there still was an important lesson I needed to learn.

In 2011, my daughter, Alana, was about ten months old when I began having heart pain and shortness of breath. There she was, not even walking yet, and I was unable to hold her or pick her up. I was afraid I was going to have a heart attack. Never before had I experienced pain in my heart. I thought about calling 911, but followed my intuition instead and contacted Tom, who thankfully answered his phone. I told him about the tightness in my heart and my inability to take a deep breath. It was getting painful, and scary.

Over the phone, Tom took a look (energetically) at my heart and saw that many people were corded (energetically) to my heart. There was no malicious intent. Just loved ones cording to my heart energetically. So he began pulling cords from the front and back of my heart. At the end of one hour, I had 90% relief. Later that evening, the pain was completely gone. I wondered to myself, "How many people end up in the emergency room because of energy cords?" So I asked Tom, and he replied, "All the time."

By now I fully believe in energy medicine. I also came to realize how important it is to know and practice ways to clear oneself. Some of us are naturally more prone than others to picking up the energy of others. The reasons for this varies.

Most the time I can clear myself now, but if something comes up that feels bigger than me, I make an appointment with a trusted, experienced energy healer.

I've continued to learn more. Energy is very powerful and can be experienced as negative, positive, or neutral. Our thoughts create our reality. In this way, we are co-creators with the Divine. We can use energy in positive ways to help ourselves heal, as in the Universal Love Meditation provided in the meditation chapter. ♦

How I Explored Alternative Medicine—Sheri M.

My health issues took me on an exploration of self-discovery as I sifted through many different healing alternatives on my path to wellness.

First, I met with a naturopathic doctor who guided me regarding nutrition, supplements, and used hands-on healing, a form of energy medicine to clear certain organs and meridians in my body. I also saw a chiropractor that helped align my neck and spine which minimized my muscular pain.

I enrolled in a yoga class at a health club but the classes were too challenging for my state of health at that time. For this reason, I created my own yoga meditation practice, customizing it to fit my needs and abilities. What began as a few yoga poses has evolved into a thirty to forty-five-minute program I do at least five times a week in the morning encompassing stretching, yoga, and deep breathing and meditation. This practice has become so beneficial that my body really misses it when I skip a day.

During this time of healing, I expressed my thoughts through journaling, a great outlet for getting my feelings and frustrations out and onto paper. This helped me to transfer all my concerns and worries in my head to paper which enabled me to sleep better.

As part of my healing journey, together with a group led by my naturopathic doctor, we traveled to Brazil to experience John of God, a world-renowned psychic surgeon who performs medical procedures and healings. While there, I received a group energy healing which was very positive and powerful. My time in Brazil further expanded my belief system about alternative ways of healing.

Then a good friend referred me to her medical intuitive. A medical intuitive is an intuitive counselor who is gifted in perceiving information concerning the human body. He or she can energetically see and "read" the inside of the body (organs, glands, blood, etc.). This work is done by intuitively scanning the body for areas of imbalance that may need alignment or treatment. Often times a medical intuitive will be able to know the connection of the energy to an emotion or the event causing the illness.

I'm grateful for the opportunity to have explored alternative medicine which has taught me ways to create and customize my own daily practice. As a result, I feel healthier, more grounded and peaceful. ◆

We now introduce you to Will, a dear friend of Angie's and a wonderful energy healer (the one who healed her sacrum issue). He shares his passion for assisting others in their healing journey and has witnessed many miracles along the way.

Witnessing Miracles—Will S.

The main reason I continue to love doing my work after thirty-five years is twofold. First, this lifetime for me is service—I am here to do God's work. As an emissary of love, I do what I can to make (at least my little corner of) the planet a better world. Secondly, my heart sings every time I witness someone creating a miracle for themselves.

I often have new clients (and old ones) come to me with similar situations: a doctor giving them a dire prognosis where they are going to die soon or face a life of suffering. My job then is simultaneously using energy healing to erase the fear and doubt, and witnessing and assisting my client in accessing a force within themselves that mobilizes the healing power of the human spirit and they transmute the death sentence into being alive and well.

I have been privileged to facilitate many of those big miracles over the years. There are also the hundreds and hundreds of times where, through my work, the client breaks through old beliefs and programs of lack and limitation that have prevented them from experiencing their true joy, abundance, and vibrant health they deserve. These are magnificent miracles because my client receives a new lease on life and often breaks free of old patterns of destruction.

In addition to my private practice over the past thirty-five years, I have worked in three different centers often seeing traumatic injuries and people in severe chronic pain. I worked in an acute rehabilitation hospital, a physical therapy center for back and spine injuries, and was the clinical director of a chronic pain program in a large hospital. Each of those positions helped hone my skills in working with clients who are suffering.

Even though it wasn't in my job description in those positions, I would frequently use my energy healing technologies to assist a patient in moving from suffering to hope to wellness. In dealing with chronic pain, chronic illness, or life-threatening disease, I learned there are many factors beyond the diagnosis influencing the present state and the eventual outcome for the individual.

It is deeply gratifying for me to watch my clients move from despair, suffering, or immense pain (both physical and emotional) to a return to a productive, healthy, and fulfilling life. For most, the journey is not an easy one and the roles I usually play are emotional and psychic healer, coach/mentor, and especially a teacher of techniques that will enable one to master what is necessary to turn their life around. I also see myself as friend and cheerleader, and the one who uses healing technology to transmute fears, beliefs, and old programs into a positive force for my client.

That sense of commitment to service I have now hasn't always been forefront of my consciousness. In the mid-seventies, I had established a successful career as a commercial advertising photographer with a studio in San Francisco. Outwardly I was doing well but my heart was no longer excited about my work. Something important was missing in my life and it bothered me deeply that I had no idea what it was. The turning point came while I was taking photographs for a massage book. I asked the author to train me in the particular deep tissue therapy he was using. The first time I touched someone with a pure healing intent my heart lit up and I was filled with joy. That began a two-year odyssey of studying various techniques of massage and acupressure followed by hypnotherapy and biofeedback and then building a successful practice in San Francisco in the early eighties.

When clients began experiencing dramatic physical and emotional healings during the sessions it became obvious that I needed to expand my knowledge of energy healing and spiritual transformation. The axiom, "When the student is ready the teacher appears," has been absolutely true in my case. Although I have taught and continue to teach many and varied healing therapies over the years, I consider myself an eternal student. Every situation and client is unique.

Entering each session I bring with me all the knowledge gained from studying many different technologies and the experience of having worked with many different physical, emotional, spiritual, and psychic challenges. My principle job in any session is to act as an intermediary between the Universal Force/God and the mind, body, and spirit of the individual I am working with. As the session progresses, I am guided by those two forces to access the proper "tools" from my "tool box" of learned technologies and experience to assist in the transformation of the presenting issue through the clearing of imbedded beliefs and programs and fears that are limiting them

Healing miracles take place in many wonderful ways. Sometimes, it involves subtle shifts in perception that result in profound shifts in one's life. At other times, the miracles are quite dramatic. Here are a few interesting cases from my years of service:

1. In 1999, a single mother in her forties was referred by another client because she was told by an orthopedic surgeon she had such severe degenerative disc disease that her only hope for living a functional life with minimal pain was a complete spinal fusion. Doctors told her she would be on heavy pain meds for the rest of her life and eventually in a wheelchair even with the surgery. She was understandably terrified. According to her opening statement to me, even with heavy medication her pain level was almost intolerable and had been for years.

At the end of the first session she sat up, gently moved her body, and said that for the first time in ten years she had no pain. The first of her surgeries scheduled for the following week was postponed to see what would happen with a few more sessions. When she arrived for the fourth session she was almost completely titrated from the pain medication and she had grown two inches. Because of a lifetime history of abuse, she had unconsciously compacted her body in an attempt to be invisible. As she released the deep emotional holding patterns, her spine literally sprung up. As of 2014, she has not had any back surgery and lives a full life.

2. This next case involves a woman in her early sixties who came to me because she was depressed and very frustrated with her life and her lack of connection with her Divine Source. It was interfering with her ability to be totally present in her relationship and life in general.

Rather than tell you what happened, I will let her words describe the result of her one session with me:

"I am writing to you to thank you again for the help you gave me last week. I have been on this path for a long, long time searching for my True Self and have not had much success. I have been a Roman Catholic, an agnostic, and an atheist. I have been a devotee of Hindu Shivaism, Tibetan Buddhism, and Native American Shamanism. I have studied Western astrology, Vedic astrology, numerology, and the tarot. I have meditated and prayed. I even pursued and obtained a Master of Arts degree in Counseling. I enjoyed myself and obtained much knowledge, but never did I feel that any kind of internal, spiritual, or emotional transformation took place. Yesterday, though, being with you and your kind, skillful facilitation changed that for me. I have finally had my first break-through. The peace I feel is something I have longed for most of my life. Thank you a million times." P. M., Napa, CA

3. The third case is about the power of the human spirit to mobilize healing forces when needed. Over the decades of doing my work, I have witnessed many people create miracles for themselves. Before coming to me, many of my clients were told some version of: there was nothing more that could be done for them medically and they needed to be at peace with the way things are or that they were going to die soon from whatever life-threatening disease they had. The blessing in this is every one of my patients chose to rally the forces within themselves to heal their body and return to a productive life instead. This is the story of one such miracle.

A young woman about thirty-six was admitted to the acute rehab hospital in which I was the director of the department of biotherapy. I was part of the team tasked with doing what we could for her rehabilitation. She had brain stem encephalitis and upon admission she was a total quadriplegic, unable to move her body at all and unable to swallow or speak. She could breathe on her own and move her head to some degree. The prognosis given to her by the doctors was that the best she could probably hope for was eventually some gross motor movement in her limbs. They didn't hold much hope for her ever swallowing again either. While the other therapies did what they could for her physically, I worked with the emotional, mental, and psychic aspects of the issue.

She had a very strong, determined spirit which made it easy to focus her energy away from the prognosis and on to the task of proving the doctors wrong. We worked five days a week on visualizing herself walking, swallowing, talking, and living a normal life. As in any such healing, there is a roller coaster of encouraging physical progress and then setbacks which have the expected emotional response. Realizing the power of emotional energy, I would use the frequent discouragement in the beginning of therapy to turn that energy into a stronger determination to heal her body. It took her over three months and she walked out of the hospital on her own, talking and swallowing normally. One month later she called me to say that she had just taken her first aerobics class again! In a later conversation, she reported how the experience was a major wakeup call and she was totally re-orienting her life and work priorities around what fulfilled her emotionally and spiritually. A far cry from the type A, driven-to-succeed personality she was prior to the onset of the disease. ◆

(Will Scott's website is www.accesslife.net.)

Below is a story written by Laurie D. who healed her back pain using a spiritual clearing modality called Spiritual Response Therapy (SRT).

Healing Back Pain with Spiritual Response Therapy —Laurie D.

Using Spiritual Response Therapy (SRT) protocol, I was able to discern that an energy of despair for me was showing up as "pressing" and "depressing" energy on my disk and creating back pain.

This despair energy that manifested as back pain was from a past life relationship showing up in this lifetime in my relationship with my husband. Once the root cause of that despair energy was identified and cleared, the back and disk symptom of pain stopped. My back continues to remain healthy, strong, and free of pain. ♦

More about SRT—Laurie D.

Now, one may ask, how do I know if a problem is rooted in a past life relationship? Or what if I do not believe in past lives of one's soul? One knows if a problem is rooted in a past life relationship by doing research using SRT procedures/protocol. If one does not believe in past lives, that is okay; with approval to do the research, the research as to root cause can be completed and benefit will be felt by the client.

I am grateful for both of these techniques that get to the root cause and naturally resolve issues presenting themselves as symptoms. There are trained, certified SRT consultants worldwide (in various languages) who are available to give you a clearing over the phone. If you're interested in learning more about SRT, go to www.spiritualresponse.com. ♦

When our energies are aligned—through meditation, prayer, our intentions—for the highest good of all concerned, amazing things happen. But we need to pay attention to those intuitive hits or impulses that may be guiding us. We need to learn to trust our intuition.

Let's open our minds and start believing in miracles. Below is a story written by Gloria. Gloria told me she has always believed in miracles, even before she had this seemingly miraculous healing.

Spontaneous Healing of Pain and Inflammation
—Gloria A.

On Wednesday morning I was getting ready to meet Angie at the Lafayette Reservoir. I didn't feel well because my ankles were incredibly swollen. Although they had been abnormally swollen for the past several weeks, they were especially big on Wednesday.

Despite my physical discomfort, I was looking forward to hearing Angie's encouraging thoughts and words. The pain and discomfort were increasing significantly as I pushed myself to walk.

Angie knew I meditated and that my spirit was strong. So she asked me what I was saying to myself (if anything) during my meditations and affirmations. I verbalized to Angie that I was saying (and thinking) that "Although my body is failing, I won't let my spirit fail."

Angie immediately pointed out the harm of the word "failing" and how that was reinforcing the pain I was feeling in my ankle and my body "failing" to get better. She suggested that I use positive words instead such as, "My body is healing and my spirit is aligned with health" so that I could attract positive energy toward my body. I repeated these words. In addition, she explained to me that sometimes we also need to disconnect from negative external energies as well as internal negative thoughts.

Her spirit was so rejuvenated and enlightened, which inspired me to reflect on myself and to distance from any thoughts and people who were not positively contributing to my life. Everything we were sharing with one another resonated so profoundly with each of us that we even experienced a moment of complete awe.

We continued our walk. Angie also taught me about energy cords. Energy cords are an energy exchange between two people where you are connected to another person by an energetic cord. You may be influencing each other in negative ways. I immediately sensed that my ex-husband was corded to my low back. So we stopped walking and I reached back to the area and firmly removed that cord.

My daughter, who has been visiting from college, was on the walk with us and was so excited to witness the power of positive energy.

By the end of our walk, I was thinking about what had just happened. Angie's energy level was particularly high and she helped me shift into a more positive frame of mind and perspective.

It was then that I realized I was completely relieved of the pain and inflammation I had felt earlier. My ankles and legs had miraculously deflated to their normal sizes. Even my leggings were baggy toward the bottom!

It has been several weeks since the walk that day and my ankles continue to be normal. The combination of Angie's energy and my intuitive action prompted by her teaching me about energy and cords, resulted in a profound physical healing for me. ◆

My Journey of the Spirit—Sheri M.

My spiritual journey got underway as a young girl when my mother taught me a simple prayer to say before going to sleep:

Dear God, thank you for being so good to me today. And please dear God, be good to my mother, my father, my brothers and everybody who I love. Thank you dear God, good night dear God, Amen. This prayer comforted me through my formative years and helped me feel connected to a greater source.

As my mother was the eldest of eight children, I grew up as part of a large extended family. I was surrounded and nurtured by a loving grandmother, aunts, uncles, and cousins.

Living in close proximity to one another, we got together often. There was the monthly family club, outings to the beach, picnics in the park, hayrides and sharing of holidays. Our annual Chanukah party was an extra special event, filled with Jewish traditions, glowing candles, gifts for the kids, and lots of love. Although my family wasn't particularly religious, Judaism served as a heart-warming tradition in my life. These family ties provided me with many fond memories through the years.

The prayer I had recited as a young girl faded into the background as I grew into my teenager years and questioned the existence of God. As a child, I had imagined God, as many children do, as a benevolent man with a long white beard, up in heaven, watching over us. This image no longer held meaning as I questioned God's existence and pondered the meaning of life. The answers to these questions would come together in later years.

I married in my early 20s and had a very conventional marriage. As the women's movement emerged, it gave me a new lens for viewing my role as a wife and mother. I could no longer live the image of a traditional housewife.

Eventually, my marriage of almost twenty-five years came to an end.

Before embarking on my new life, I felt compelled to go back to my family roots. I journeyed to Budapest, Hungary, with my father who, at the age of eighty-three, had not returned to his homeland since his twenties. I searched out where my ancestors came from, explored the neighborhoods and haunts where my father grew up, spent hours locating my paternal grandmother's grave, and ventured deep into the Carpathian mountains of Romania to track down my maternal grandmother's village.

Little by little the history of my ancestry came together and I felt more connected to my past and more in touch with who I was in the present.

Shortly after returning home from Europe and finalizing my divorce, I contracted Lyme disease from a tick bite in my garden in Lafayette, California. Traditional Western medical doctors weren't yet informed about this disease, so I began to explore other options. This opened my eyes to alternative and complementary medicine. As a seeker and an avid learner, I explored various healing modalities and what I came to learn changed my life in profound ways.

I took numerous courses and studied books about the chakra system, meditation, intuition, and energy medicine. One of the first books I read was Shirley MacLaine's The Camino, A Journey of the

Spirit, a challenging pilgrimage that gradually gives way to a voyage of the soul. I realized that I was on a voyage of my own soul.

I began to take a more global view of what a belief in God meant to me. I came to believe in a "generic spirituality" where the God source is the same for all humanity, regardless of the religion you follow, and where all religions are viewed as valid paths to God.

As I've expanded my interpretation of God to include Spirit, Higher Power and Universal Source, Judaism continues to be an important part of my life. My current feeling is that there is an energy that I can connect to and know that I'm supported by it. This has been an essential part of my healing journey.

I've come to understand that I'm here on earth to learn lessons and make a contribution to others. As I align with this purpose and get in the flow of this energy, it becomes easier to get in touch with my inner healer. Each of us has the opportunity to connect with this energy within and get help with whatever needs healing in our lives. ♦

My Spiritual Journey—Angie L.

Growing up as a young girl in South Dakota, I intuitively sensed the presence of God. Faith wasn't something I had to work at. It was just there.

In middle school and high school, I went to church by myself and sometimes took my best friend, Shelley, with me. I enjoyed the tradition of worshiping, singing, praying and being in community.

By my late 20s, my sense of religion evolved into a broader, more spiritual, all-encompassing belief system. I began to resonate with teachings that transcended a particular religious denomination and learned that each of us is magnificent...a brilliant, unique emanation of the Divine. That there is a power, a presence and a love within each of us that we can rely upon.

I learned about Marianne Williamson (*A Return to Love*) and became a student of *A Course in Miracles* where I studied the concept that in any given moment and in every decision there's an opportunity to choose love over fear.

I worked with a trained coach to learn Transcendental Meditation, known as TM. I was assigned a mantra, and began a meditation practice. I enjoyed the benefits of focusing on a mantra and liked how it quieted my mind. Throughout my life, I've had a strong desire to know myself spiritually, to be balanced emotionally and be well and strong physically.

The Bay Area intuitive-energy schools I attended teach about "owning your own space" and getting free of energetic cords. Some people choose to keep cords in place while others choose to be free of them. Once you are aware of them, it's a choice. Carrying energy that's not yours can lower your vibration and disrupt your energy field, influencing all aspects of your being.

I learned tools to become more intimately familiar with my energy body, which is an aspect of my spiritual body. I learned to connect to the wisdom contained within my body, the "smart" body or innate body, as it is referred to.

My body allows me to tune into my internal guidance system for decision making. I used muscle testing for years (getting yes or no responses by leaning forward or leaning back) before working with a pendulum. Then I used a pendulum for about 10 years to receive guidance and help me make decisions. Eventually, I didn't need either to know or to feel into my answers and higher guidance.

Our body carries a wealth of information if we tune in and pay attention. Our body will inform us if a relationship, a job, a book, a particular food or supplement is right for us, or not. No matter how big or small the question is, the body knows the answer.

The more I learned to keep my energy field clear, the more I can tune into to my own information and guidance and trust it. This skill has taken me years to cultivate. I'm grateful for the journey.

Meanwhile, as I developed awareness of my body and my energy field, I also strengthened my connection with God and my angels. I learned from Doreen Virtue's angel books that angels only have permission to intervene in life or death situations. So if we need help in other areas, any area, we must ask and give them permission to assist us.

This has been a profound experience for me—to ask and to receive. If I need help balancing the energy of a relationship and bringing more harmony to it, they help. If I'm struggling to sleep well, I ask for help and get it. If I need help manifesting an important intention, I receive it. Maybe not always in my timeline, but eventually, it happens.

Trust and faith help us relax, less go of worry and stress, which help us stay healthier, longer. Our spiritual connection gives us the strength to take on life's challenges head on, with confidence. Whatever is going on, there's a feeling of being taken care of, no matter what. This feeling gives me inner peace that all is well, despite appearances. A knowingness that everything is unfolding as it should. I let go and trust.

I overcame a debilitating form of rheumatoid arthritis and put to rest years of suffering with severe psoriasis. Whatever the struggle, whatever the diagnosis, know that healing is possible. No matter what anyone else says. ♦

GLOSSARY OF
ALTERNATIVE HEALTH CARE METHODS

Below are definitions of health care methods we want to highlight. There are hundreds more out there but these are the ones we feel most people would get value from trying.

- **Acupressure.** Stimulates the flow of vital energy, or chi, circulating along the body's meridians thereby influencing the functioning of certain internal organs. By applying thumb and fingertip pressure, specific symptoms are relieved and balance is restored to the entire body. Effective for treating stress, sciatica, arthritis, headaches, fatigue, and general irritability.

- **Acupuncture.** The art of inserting fine needles at specific points along the body's meridians to stimulate, disperse, and regulate the flow of chi (energy). Acupuncture is used to relieve symptoms, especially pain relief, as well as to promote general health and well-being.

- **Alexander Technique.** In this form of movement education, practitioners use gentle hands on guidance, and lead the client through a series of lessons designed to improve postural habits, increase freedom of movement, and reduce physical tension.

- **Ayurvedic Medicine.** Focuses on disease prevention by maintaining the body's natural equilibrium through dietary changes, yoga, meditation, herbs, massage, and possibly chanting depending on one's nature or dosha (body type): vata, pitta and kapfa.

- **Bach Flower Remedies/Essences.** Flower essences administered in liquid form improve one's state of well-being by eliminating negative emotions.

- **Bodywork.** A general term used to describe any type of manual, manipulative healing modality that aims to restore health of body, mind, and spirit. Some examples include massage, craniosacral therapy, and acupressure.

- **Cellular Memory Release Therapy.** This is a self-help synthesis that combines practical ancient Tibetan corrections with the latest brain integration techniques that became available after decades of research on the brain and human programming. Cellular memory release is a very simple and, yet, effective way to treat emotional and electrical imbalances in the body. This is a method of re-patterning self-sabotaging behavior as you access files that were written in the past and are affecting your present.

• **Chakra Balancing.** Based on the oriental wisdom that the body has seven main energy centers along the spine that absorb and emit life force. Each chakra governs an area of the body together with specific emotional issues. Poor health can result when blockages occur due to mental and emotional issues, poor nutrition, drugs, and injury.

• **Chinese Medicine.** A holistic perspective on health and illness which treats the relationship of a symptom to the person as a whole. Traditional Chinese medicine encompasses a vast range of therapies including acupuncture, herbs, bodywork, exercise, and diet.

• **Chiropractic Treatment.** Relieves pressure on the nervous system with precise adjustments to the spinal segments or to individual vertebrae. Structural alignment can alleviate a myriad of symptoms.

• **Colon Hydrotherapy.** This therapy cleanses the colon through gentle water infusions. Colonics are recommended for ailments such as constipation, psoriasis, acne, allergies, headaches, and are used for general health balance.

• **Color Therapy.** The body responds at a cellular level to specific frequencies of colored light applied to the skin at acupuncture points. This therapy is effective in balancing the body and healing various physical and mental disorders such as depression.

• **Craniosacral Therapy.** This specialized treatment focuses on the craniosacral system comprised of the brain, spinal cord, meninges, cranial bones, and sacrum. This craniosacral system contains fluid, which moves with slight but perceptible rhythmic fluctuation. By using gentle pressure, tension in the body is reduced and balance is restored to the central nervous system.

• **Crystal Healing.** An alternative technique that employs stones and crystals for strengthening the body and resolving issues and patterns. It is a process of bringing energy fields into alignment.

• **(EFT) Emotional Freedom Technique.** Based on the energy meridians used in acupuncture. Simple tapping with the fingertips is used to input energy onto specific meridians on the head and chest while thinking about a specific problem and voicing positive affirmations. This combination of tapping and voicing works to clear the emotional block, restoring your mind and body's balance.

• **Energy Healing.** Imbalances in the physical body first develop in the subtle energy bodies such as our aura and chakras. Our energy systems become out of balance primarily through exposure to the stresses–of day-to-day life. Balancing them through various techniques (for example, SRT, EFT, NET, Reiki, etc.) enables the body's mechanisms to function at optimal levels thus preventing disease; this accelerates the healing process.

• **Feldenkrais.** Movement therapy that identifies how we use or misuse our bodies and the subsequent effect on health. It corrects poor posture and movement habits, and is useful in the treatment of arthritis, back pain, muscle injuries, and physical problems including spasticity, stress, and tension.

• **Five Rhythms.** A form of free dance stemming from the work of Gabrielle Roth. The five rhythms, Flowing, Staccato, Chaos, Lyrical, and Stillness form the Wave, a dance form that crosses the boundaries between art, therapy, Shamanic healing, and spiritual impulse.

• **Guided Imagery.** A gentle but powerful technique that focuses and directs the imagination. Imagery has the built-in capacity to deliver multiple layers of complex, encoded messages by way of simple symbols and metaphors.

• **Healing Touch.** A program of energy techniques developed by a nurse, Janet Mentgen, in 1989. Healing Touch is used to accelerate wound healing, relieve pain, promote relaxation, and prevent illness.

• **Hakomi Therapy.** Integrates Eastern spiritual traditions with a unique Western body-centered psychology to bring core beliefs which shape our lives and relationships into consciousness for possible transformation. This therapy is based on the principles of mindfulness, nonviolence, and the unity of mind and body.

• **Herbal Medicine.** Herbal remedies are given in tinctures, decoctions, infusions, compresses, poultices, capsules, lozenges, or ointments to treat illness or enhance the body's ability to function efficiently.

• **Homeopathy.** Uses minute doses of the substance causing an illness to cure the same illness. In theory the "remedies" stimulate a person's immune systems and help the body heal itself. Homeopathy can be used to treat short-term illnesses or chronic ailments.

• **Hypnosis.** In a therapeutic environment, hypnosis accesses the subconscious mind for the purpose of enhancing, changing, or eliminating behaviors.

• **Iridology.** A person's state of health or the presence of disease are reflected in and can be diagnosed by examining the patterns of the eye.

• **Jin Shin Jyutsu.** An ancient art of harmonizing the life energy in the body by the balancing of combinations of energy centers.

• **Kinesiology.** The study of anatomy, physiology, and mechanics of body movement. Also known as "muscle testing," it can be used to determine the root cause of a condition. Practitioners view the body as an intelligent computer. Through kinesiology they can identify the problem area and treat it.

• **Massage Therapy.** The primary goal is to encourage relaxation, healing, and well-being. Massage is useful in the treatment of anxiety, back pain, cancer, circulation problems, colic, depression, headaches, heart disorders, high blood pressure, hyperactivity, insomnia, sinusitis, and tension.

• **Medical-Osteopathy.** Osteopathy is an established and recognized system of diagnosis and treatment, which puts its main emphasis on the structural and functional integrity of the body. It is distinctive by the fact that it recognizes that much of the pain and disability that we suffer from stems from abnormalities in the function of the body structure as well as damage caused to it by disease.

• **Meditation.** A mental technique for deep relaxation, meditation helps to focus and calm the mind. It may be used to heal the body, quiet the mind, and provide a sense of inner balance.

• **Mindfulness Based Stress Reduction.** This form of meditation cultivates greater awareness of the unity of mind and body, as well as unconscious thoughts, feelings, and behaviors that can undermine emotional, physical, and spiritual health.

- **NAET.** A holistic, non-invasive treatment used in eliminating food and environmental allergies. NAET stands for Nambudripad's allergy elimination technique and is a combination of Western sciences, kinesiology, and chiropractic and was developed to specialize exclusively in the diagnosis and treatment of allergies.
- **Naturopathic Medicine.** This health care system emphasizes prevention, treatment, and optimal health through the use of therapeutic methods and substances that encourage individuals' inherent self-healing process. The practice combines acupuncture, nutrition, herbalism, homeopathy, osteopathy, and hydrotherapy.
- **Neuro-Emotional Technique (NET).** A holistic approach that combines traditional Chinese medicine, chiropractic, and applied kinesiology that finds and removes unresolved "negative emotional blocks," toxins in the body, and deficiencies in nutrition.
- **Pilates Method.** An exercise system focused on improving flexibility and strength for the total body without building bulk. It is a series of controlled movements engaging body and mind, performed on specifically designed exercise apparatus and supervised by extensively trained teachers.
- **Pranic Healing.** A simple, powerful, and effective no-touch energy healing technique. It is based on the fundamental principal that the body is a "self-repairing" living entity that possesses the innate ability to heal itself. Pranic healing works on the principal that the healing process is accelerated by increasing the life force or vital energy on the affected part of the physical body.
- **Reflexology.** A system based on the principle that the whole body has reflex points in the feet and hands which can be stimulated by massage to correct disorders in the corresponding parts of the body.
- **Reiki.** Japanese word for universal life force. It is a form of energy therapy where practitioners transmit energy by a light touch, placing their hands gently in specific positions on the body. It is effective for many physical, emotional, mental, and spiritual conditions.
- **Rolfing.** A form of structural integration using deep tissue manipulation designed to balance the body physically and energetically and release embedded emotional patterns.

• **Self Muscle Testing.** An alternative healing diagnostic tool that allows one to ask the body yes or no questions. It works with the idea that a positive association or "yes" strengthens the muscles, while a negative association or "no" weakens them.

• **Sound Therapy.** States of well-being and consciousness have corresponding frequency patterns. Sound therapy applies acoustic energy as voice tones or music in an ambient environment.

• **Spiritual Response Therapy (SRT).** SRT is a step-by-step process of researching the subconscious mind and the soul records to discover and release hidden subconscious blocks to health, happiness, and spiritual growth using thirty-two charts, one's intuition, and a pendulum.

• **Touch for Health Therapy.** Through specialized kinesiology, the functioning and condition of the skeletal, muscular, circulatory, endocrine, and nervous systems is accessed and evaluated. This information is then used to identify where the mind-body requires improvement and to restore the natural energy flow and movement to the body.

• **Tragar Therapy.** Uses light, gentle, rhythmic, passive movements which facilitates the release of deep-seated physical and mental patterns. It is effective for treating musculoskeletal injuries and the effects of neuromuscular and stress related disorders.

• **Vibrational Medicine.** Practitioners use electric, magnetic, sonic, acoustic, microwave, light/color, and energy frequency devices to screen for and treat health conditions by detecting and correcting imbalances in the body's energy field.

• **Watsu.** An ancient form of Japanese massage called Zin Shiatsu is a sequence of gentle movement and stretches, as you are held in warm water.

• **Yoga.** Combines postures with breath work to stimulate the flow of subtle energies in the body to clear and activate chakras, thereby raising your energy. Yoga is widely practiced for health and relaxation.

References

Chapter 1 Our Journeys Back to Health
1. Jason Theodosakis, MD, MS, MPH, FACPM and Sheila Buff, The Arthritis Cure, St. Martins Griffin, (2004)

Chapter 2 America's Health Today
1. Trogdon, J. G., Cohen, "Annual medical spending attributable to obesity" (2009). *Health Affairs,* 28(5), w808–w817"
2. Ligouri, A. Mozumdar, "Persistent increase of prevalence of metabolic syndrome among US adults," American Diabetes Assn. (2011)
3. Mark Hyman, MD, *The Blood Sugar Solution,* Little, Brown & Company (2012)
4. Steven Nissen, MD, "Clock's Ticking: Decreasing Cardiac and Stroke Death Rate," Cleveland Clinic (2013)
5. www.acscan.org
6. www.abcnews.go.com/GMA/AmericanFamily/storyid=12
7. www.medicalnewtoday.com/articles/270202.phpwww.
8. www.cdc.gov
9. www.diabetes.org
10. www.cancer.gov/about-cancer/understading/statistics,

Chapter 3 Reasons for Our Declining Health
1. William Davis, MD, *Wheat Belly,* Rodale, (2011)
2 Jordan S. Rubin, *The Makers Diet,* Destiny Image Publisher (2005)
3. Rosane Oliveira, DVM, PhD, "The Straight Truth About Organic," UC Davis Integrative Medicine (2015)
4. Johnson, R. K., "Dietary Sugars Intake and Cardiovascular Health," American Heart Association, Circulation, (2009)
5. www.ucdintegrativemedicine.com
6. www.wiley.com, *The Journal of the Science of Food and Agriculture* (2017)
7.www.health.harvard.edu/blog,thelongthelongoodbyefdarulingwilleliminatetransfat sfromusfoods (2015)

Chapter 4 Mindful Eating
www.drweil.com/diet-nutrition/food-safety/what-does-mindful-eating-really-mean/2014

Chapter 5 Foods That Heal
1. Maureen Salaman, *Foods That Heal: Prevent or Reverse More Than 100 Common Ailments,* Stratford Publishing (1989)
2. Bauman, Edward, M.Ed., PhD. *Eating for Health: Your Guide to Vitality & Optimal Health,* Bauman (2008)
3. Michael Lara, MD, *The Pharmacy in Your Kitchen* (2017)
4. Cherie Calbom, MS and Maureen Keane, MS, *Juicing for Life*, Avery Trade (1991)
5. Marc David, *Nourishing Wisdom*, Random House (1991)

Chapter 6 GMOs and Organic Foods
1. Jeffrey Smith Documentary: *GMO Trilogy Seeds of Deception,* Chelsea Green Publishing (2003)
2. Weston A. Price Foundation "Wise Traditions in Food and Farming," *Healing Arts* magazine, (2014)
3. Maria Rosedale, *Organic Manifesto: How Organic Food Can Heal Our Planet, Feed the World, and Keep Us Safe,* Rodale (2010)
4. www.organicconsumers.org
5. www.ushealthworks.com/blog/index.php/ "have-you-loaded-up-on-your-bioflavonoids-today" (2012)

Chapter 7 Beans, Beans
http://beaninstitute.com/recipes/bean-referne-chart

Chapter 8 Our Love Affair with Coffee and Chocolate
1. Mercola.com, "The Surprising Benefits of Drinking Coffee" (2011)
2. Melanie King, *Tea, Coffee & Chocolate: How We Fell in Love with Caffeine* (2015)

Chapter 9 A Story That Supports How Food Heals
1. Rausch "Nutrition and Academic Performance in School-Age Children," *Journal of Nutrition & Food Sciences* (2013)
2. Daphne Miller MD, *The Jungle Effect: Healthiest Diets from Around the World—Why They Work and How to Make Them Work for You*, Harper (2011)
3. Pure Facts DVD: *Impact of Fresh, Healthy Foods on Learning and Behavior: Roadmap to Healthy Foods in School,* Natural Press (2002)
4. www.feingoldorg/PF/wisconsin

Chapter 10 Food Allergies and Food Sensitivities
1. Elizabeth Gordon, *Simply Allergy—Free: Quick and Easy Recipes for Every Night of the Week,* Roman & Littlefield (2013)

2. Caroline M. Sutherland, *The Body Knows Diet: Cracking the Weight-Loss Code*, Hay House, Inc. (2005)

3. James Braly MD, *Hidden Food Allergies: The Essential Guide to Uncovering Hidden Food Allergies-And Achieving Permanent Relief*, Basic Health Education, Inc. (2009)

4. "The Art and Science of Healthy Living" *Alternative Medicine* magazine (2005)

5. Phyllis Austin, *Food Allergies Made Simple: The Complete Manual for Diagnosis, Treatment, and Prevention of Food Allergies*, Family Health Publications (1985)

6. www.carolinesutherland.com

7. www.naet.com

Chapter 11 Gluten Sensitivities

1. Vickki & Richard Peterson, D.C., C.C.N, *The Gluten Effect: How Innocent Wheat is Ruining your Health*, True Health Publishing (2009)

2. William Davis MD, *Wheat Belly*, Rodale (2011)

3. John G. Herron, *The Gut Health Protocol: A Natural Approach to Healing SIBO, Intestinal Candida, GERD, Gastritis, and Other Gut Health Issues*, Eagle Stock Publishing (2016)

4. www.gfrecipes.com

5. www.celiac.org

6. www.gluten.net

7. www.celiaccentral.org

8. www.celiac.com

9. *Living Without* magazine (2011)

Chapter 12 Dairy and Other Sensitivities

1. JJ Virgin, *The Virgin Diet*, Harlequin (2012)

2. *Living Without* magazine Oct. (2010)

3. Caroline Sutherland, *The Body Knows* Diet, Hay House Inc. (2005)

4. Gary Null, MD, *Food-Mood-Body Connection*, Seven Stories Press (2000)

5. Russell Blaylock, MD, *Excitoxins: The Taste That Kills*, Health Press (1997)

6. Caroline Sutherland, *The Body Knows Diet: Cracking the Weightloss Code*, Hay House (2008)

7. www.bodyecology.com

Chapter 13 Sugar and Its Many Disguises

1. Ann Louise Gittleman, PhD, CNS, *Get the Sugar Out Sugar: 501 Simple Ways to Cut the Sugar Out of any Diet*, Three Rivers Press (2008)

2. Robert H. Lustig, MD, *The Real Truth About Sugar*, River City eBooks, (2011)

3. Joseph Mercola, MD, and Kendra Degen Pearsall, ND, *Sweet Deception*, Joseph Mercola (2006)

4. Nancy Appleton, PhD, *Lick the Sugar Habit*, Avery (2001)

5. Connie Bennett, CHHC with Stephen T. Sinatra, MD, *Sugar Shock: How Sweets and Simple Carbs Can Derail Your Life—and How You Can Get Back on Track,* Berkeley Books, (2006)

6. www.health.com: Nutrition 2017)

7. www.fasttrackkicksugar.com

Chapter 14 Artificial Sugars and Healthy Alternatives

1. Russell L. Blaylock, MD, *Excitotoxins: The Taste That Kills* Health Press (1994)

2. Connie Bennett, C.H.H.C., *Sugar Shock,* Berkley Books, (2007)

3. Emory Univ., CDC and Prevention, "Sugar lowers LDL," *Journal American Medical Association* (2013)

4. www.truthaboutslenda.com

5. www.SplendaExosed.com

6. www.naturalnews.com 2006

7. www.rodalesorganiclife.com/food/best-and-worst

Chapter 15 Inflammation and Chronic Disease

1. Jack Challem, *The Inflammation Syndrome*, John Wiley and Sons, (2010)

2. Julie Daniluk, *Meals That Heal Inflammation*, Daniluk Consulting (2011)

3. Nancy Appleton, PhD. *Stopping Inflammation: Relieving the Cause of Degenerative Disease,* Square One (2005)

4. Leonard Saputo, MD, *Boosting Immunity: Creating Wellness Naturally,* New World Library (2002)

5. Deepak Chopra, *Ageless Body, Timeless Mind: The Quantum Alternative to Growing Old*, Harmony Books (1993)

Chapter 16 Acid Alkaline, Candida, and Enzymes

1. Theodore A. Baroody, *Alkalize or Die: Superior Health Through Proper Alkaline-Acid Balance,* Holographic Health Press (2015)

2. Robert O. Young, and Shelley Redford Young, *The pH Miracle: Balance Your Diet, Reclaim Your Health,* Warner Books (2010)

3. Istvan Fazeka, *The Alkalizing Diet*, A.R.E. Press (2005)

4. William G. Crook, *The Yeast Connection Handbook: How Yeasts Can Make You Feel "sick all over" and the Steps You Need to Take to Regain Your Health,* Professional Books, Inc. (2002)

5. Sally Fallon, *Nourishing Traditions,* New Trends Publishing (2001)

6. www.livescience.com/45145-how-do-enzymes-work.html

7. WorldHealthOrganization:www.who.int/foodsafety/fs_management/en/probiotic_guidelines.pdf, (2002)

8. Edward Howell, MD, www.enzymesinc.com/enzyme-pioneer-dr-edward-howell.html

Chapter 17 Arthritis

1. Rona Zoltan, MD, *Rheumatoid Arthritis -Decrease or Reverse Symptoms Naturally*, Natural Health Guide, Alive books (2002)
2. Rona Zoltan, MD, *Osteoarthritis—Treat and Reverse Joint Pain Naturally*, Natural Health Guide, Alive Books (2002)
3. Jason Theodosakis, MD, *The Arthritis Cure: The Medical Miracle That Can Halt, Reverse, and may Even Cure Osteoarthritis*, St Martin's Griffin (2004)
4. www.arthritis.org
5.www.mayoclinic.org/diseases/conditions/arthritis/symptoms-causes/

Chapter 18 Healthy Brain, Happy You

1. David Perlmutter, MD, & Alberto Villoldo, *Power Up Your Brain: The Neuroscience of Enlightenment*, Hay House (2011)
2. Deepak Chopra, MD, & Rudolph E. Tanzi, PhD, *Super Brain: Unleashing the Explosive Power of Your Mind to Maximize Health, Happiness, and Spiritual Well-Being*, Three Rivers Press (2012)
3. Datis Kharrazian, DHSc, DC, MS, *Why Isn't My Brain Working?: A Revolutionary Understanding of Brain Decline and Effective Strategies to Recover Your Brain Health*, Elephant Press (2013)
4. Weil, Andrew, MD, *Spontaneous Happiness: A New Path to Emotional Well-Being*, Hodder & Stoughton (2015)
5. Fotuhi M, Lubinski B, Riloff T, Trullinger M, Ghasemi M "Brain Fitness Program for Treatment of Cognitive Impairment in Elderly." *JSM Alzheimer's Dis Related Dementia* 1(1): 1002 (2014)
6. Alzheimer's Association, *The Healthy Brain Initiative: A National Public Health Road Map to Maintaining Cognitive Health*: Chicago, IL (2007)
7. James De Gordon, MD, www.achievingoptimalhealthconference.com/speakers
8. Majid Fotuhi, MD & Christina Breda Antoniadesj Boost Your Brain: The New Art and Science Behind Enhanced Brain Performance, Harper One (2014)
9. Mark George, MD, National Institutes of Health
https://ajp.psychiatryonline.org/doi/pdf/10.1176/ajp.152.3.341
10. www.amenclinics.com

Chapter 19 Gut-Brain Connection
1. Majid Fotuhi & Christina Breda Antoniadesj, *Boost Your Brain: The New Art and Science Behind Enhanced Brain Performance*, Harper One (2014)
2. Teri Arranga, *Bugs, Bowels, and Behavior: The Groundbreaking Story of the Gut-Brain Connection*, Sky Horse Publishing (2013)

3. Lawrence Friedman, MD, *The Sensitive Gut,* Harvard Health Publications (2012)
4. *The Gut Brain Connection* HEALTHbeat Archive
5. James Greenblat, MD, "Gut Feelings, The Future of Psychiatry May be Inside Your Stomach: The Right Combination of Stomach Microbes Could be Crucial for a Healthy Mind," *The Verge,* Science Features (2013)

Chapter 20 Cancer—Part 1
1. Kelly A. Turner, PhD, *Radical Remission: Surviving Cancer at All Odds,* Harper One (2015)
2. Patrick Quillin, *Beating Cancer with Nutrition,* Nutrition Times Press, Inc. (2005)
3. Rosch, P.J. "Stress and Cancer," in Cooper, CL ed. *Psychosocial Stress and Cancer*, John Wiley & Sons (1984)
4. Dean Ornish, MD, "Healthy Living Halts Disease," UCSF News Center, (2013)
5. www.larc.fr/l International Agency for Research on Cancer, *Journal of the National Cancer Institute* (2013)
6. TinrinChew, OncologyDietician, www.youtube.comn/watch?y=E6y1HD-LrDQ
7. www.researchgate.net, Harvard Report on Cancer Prevention, (2017) www
8. www.cspinet.org/eating-healthy/chical-cuisine, Center for Science in the Public Interest, Chemical Cuisine
9. T. Colin Campbell, PhD, *The China Study,* Ben Bella Books, (2016)
10. www.cdc.gov
11. www.pcrm.org
12. www.berkeleywellness.com/13ways-cut-cancer-risk (2017)

Chapter 21 Cancer—Part 2
1. Kelly A. Turner, PhD. *Radical Remission, The Nine Key Factors That Can Make a Real Difference*, Harper One (2015)
2. *What Doctors Don't Tell You* Journal Magazine (April 2014)
3. www.burzynskiclinic.com
4. www.burzyskimovie.com, *Cancer Is Serious Business*
5. www.gerson.org,
6. www.CaringBridge.org
7. http://driversforsurvivors.org

Chapter 22 Cancer Recovery Stories

Chapter 23 Diabetes
1. Mark Hyman, MD, *The Blood Sugar Solution: The Ultra Healthy Program for Losing Weight, Preventing Disease, and Feeling Great Now!* Little Brown & Company (2012)

2. Maureen Keane, MS and Daniella Chace, MD, *What to Eat If You Have Diabetes: Healing Foods That Help Control Your Blood Sugar*, McGraw Hill (2007)

3. C. Leight Broadhurst, PhD, *Prevent, Treat and Reverse Diabetes, Alive Books* (2002)

4. Neal Barnard MD, *Program for Reversing Diabetes: Scientifically Proven System for Reducing Diabetes Without Drugs,* Rodale Wellness (2017)

5. www.Drrosedale.com, *Insulin and Its Metabolic Affects,* (2011)

6. Olubukola Ajala-Patrick English Jonathan Pinkney, *The American Journal of Clinical Nutrition,* Vol. 97, March (2013)

Chapter 24 Good Fats, Bad Fats

1. Nina Teicholz, T*he Big Fat Surprise*: *Why Butter, Meat & Cheese Belong in a Healthy Diet,* Simon & Schuster (2014)

2. Ann Louise Gittleman, PhD, *The New Fat Flush Plan,* McGraw Hill (2017)

3. Udo Erasmus, *Fats that Heal Fats that Kill: The Complete Guide to Fats, Oils, cholesterol and Human Health*, Alive Books (1993)

4. Andrew Weil, *Spontaneous Healing: How to Discover and Enhance Your Body's Natural Ability to Maintain and Heal Itself,* Ballantine Book (2000)

5. www.FDA.gov

6. www.proteinpower.com/drmike/2010/04/04/dining-out-and-bad-fats/

7. www.mercola.com/nutritionplan/beginner_fats.htm

8. www.wellandgood.com/...china-study-cheat-sheet-10-things-you-need-to-know

Chapter 25 Heart Disease

1. Weston A. Price Foundation, *Wise Traditions in Food, Farming and the Healing Arts (*2013)

2. Julie Daniluk, RHN, *Meals That Heal Inflammation: Embrace Healthy Living and Eliminate Pain, One Meal at a Time,* Daniluk Consulting (2011)

3. David Evans, *Cholesterol and Saturated Fat Prevent Heart Disease: Evidence from 101 Scientific Papers*, Grosvenor House Publishing Ltd. (2012)

4. Gary Taubes, *Good Calories, Bad Calories: Fats, Carbs, and the Controversial Science of Diet and Health,* Random House (2007)

5. *The Journal of the American Medical Association* (2012)

6. CNN: Dr. Sanjay Gupta's Report: "The Last Heart Attack" (2012)

7. www.sevencountriesstudy.com/about-the-study/investigators/ancel-keys/

8. www.nutritionstudies.org/the-china-study

9. Paul Ridker, MD, "How Common is Residual Inflammatory Risk?" *Circulation Research,* (2017)

10. Dwight Lundell, MD, & Todd R. Nordstrom, *The Cure for Heart Disease: Truth Will Save a Nation,* Publishing Intellect, (2011)

11. C. Norman Shealy and Carolyn Miss, The Creation of Health: The Emotional, Psychological, and Spiritual Responses That Promote Health and Healing, Three Rivers Press, (1998)

12. The American Journal of Clinical Nutrition, "Saturated fat, carbohydrate, and cardiovascular disease", https://academic.oup.com/ajcn/article abstract/91/3/502/4597078

13. www.atkins.com/.../paleo-and-atkins-how-the-diets-stack-up-with-one-another (2016)

14. www. Publichealth.llu.edu/Adventist-health-studies, (2016)

15. www.nejm.org/primary-prevention-of-cardiovascular -disease-with-a-mediterranean-diet, (2013)

16. Bruce Lipton, MD, www.brucelipton.com/resource/interview/romp-through-the-quantum-field

17. International Agency for Research on Cancer https://www.tandfonline.com/doi/abs/10.1080/10942912.2017.1375514

Chapter 26 IBS and IBD

1. Heather Van Vorous, *Eating For IBS*, Marlowe & Co. (2000)

2. Jill Sklar, *The First Year: Crohn's Disease & Colitis*: *An Essential Guide for the Newly Diagnosed*, Avalon (2007)

3. Jordan Rubin, *The Maker's Diet*: *The 40-Day Health Experience That Will Change Your Life Forever,* Destiny Image Publishers (2013)

4. Elaine Gottschall, MS, *Breaking the Vicious Cycle: Intestinal Health Through Diet,* Kirkton Press, Ltd. (1994)

5. Aglaée Jacob M.S. R.D. and Ray Sylvester, *Digestive Health with REAL Food: A Practical Guide to an Anti-Inflammatory, Nutrient Dense Diet for IBS & Other Digestive Issues,* Paleo Media Group, (2013)

6. www.helpforibs.com

Chapter 27 Leaky Gut Syndrome

1. John O. A. Pagano, *One Cause, Many Ailments: Leaky Gut Syndrome: What It Is and How It May Be Affecting Your Health,* A.R.E. Press (2008)

2. Wade Mifan, *Leaky Gut Syndrome: The Ultimate Cure Guide for How to Fix Your Leaky Gut Through A Leaky Gut Diet,* Wade Mifan (2015)

3. John G. Herron, *The Gut Protocol: A Natural Approach to Healing SIBO, Intestinal Candida, GERD, Gastritis, and Other Gut Health Issues,* Eagle Stock Publishing (2014)

Chapter 28 Obesity and Achieving Your Ideal Weight

1. Caroline Sutherland, *The Body Knows Diet: Cracking the Weightloss Code,* Hay House (2008)

2. JJ Virgin, *The Virgin Diet: Why Food Intolerance is the Real Cause of Weight Gain,* Harlequin (2012)

3. Anne Louise Gittleman, PhD, C.N.S., *The Fat Flush Plan: The Breakthrough Detox Diet,* McGraw Hill (2016)

4. Robert H. Lustig MD, *Fat Chance: Beating the Odds Against Sugar, Processed Food, Obesity, and Disease,* Penguin Group (2013)

5. Mark Hyman, MD, *The Blood Sugar Solution: The Ultra Healthy Program for Losing Weight, Preventing Disease, and Feeling Great Now!* Little, Brown & Co. (2014)

Chapter 29 Toxins in Our Home and Environment

1. Myron Wence, MD, and Dave Wence, *The Healthy Home: Simple Truths to Protect Your Family from Hidden Household Dangers,* Vanguard Press (2011)

2. Lorenzo Guaia, *The Microwaves in the Pot: Investigation of Alterations in Foods and Substances in the Microwave Ovens,* Centro Studi Luceora (2014)

3. Saputo, Leonard, MD, *A Return to Healing: Radical Health Care Reform and the Future of Medicine,* Origin Press (2009)

4. Anahad O'Connor, "The Claim: Microwave Ovens Kill Nutrients in Food," *N.Y. Times* (2006)

5. www.mercuryundercover.com

6. www.toxicteeth.org

7. www.doctorsaputo.com/a/vicki-s-corner

8. www.ewg.org/reports/skindeep

9. www.fda.gov/MedicalDevices/DentalProducts/DentalAmalgam/ucm171094

10. www.pesticideinfo.org

Chapter 30 Electromagnetic Radiation

1. James Chappell, "Avoiding EMF in the Home—Some Simple Guidelines," *Dromenon Design* (2002)

2. Thomas Rau, MD, "Electromagnetic Load, A hidden Factor in Many Illnesses," Electric Magnetic Health Blog, (2009)

3. Chris Woollams, M.A., "Cell phones and Brain Tumors—15 Reasons for Concern" *Integrated Cancer and Oncology News* (2009)

4. Anne Louise Gittleman *Zapped: Why Your Cell Phone Shouldn't Be Your Alarm Clock* and *1,268 Ways to Outsmart the Hazards of Electronic Pollution,* Harper one, (2011)

5. Devra Davis, PhD, MPH. *Disconnect—the Truth About Cell Phone Radiation,* Writers House (2013)

6. Thomas Rau, MD, "Electromagnetic Load, A hidden Factor in Many Illnesses'', Electric Magnetic Health Blog (2009)

7. Paul J. Rosch, MD, "Bioelectro Magnetic and Subtle Energy Medicine, The Interface Between Mind and Matter," *Annals of the N.Y. Academy of Sciences* (2009)

8. www.bioinitiative.org

9. www.electromagnetichealth.org

10. www.magneticpulser.us/Dr_Robert_Becker.html

11. www.fcc.gov/general/specific-absorption-rate-sar-cellular-telephones

12. www.giawellness.com

13. www.environmentalhealthtrust.org

Chapter 31 Emotions and Health

1. Nick Ortner, *The Tapping Solution: A Revolutionary System for Stress-Free Living* Hay House, Inc. (2013)

2. Bradley Nelson, M.D., *The Emotion Code*, Wellness, Unmasked Publishing, (2007)

3. Andrew Weil, MD, *Spontaneous Happiness,* Hodder & Stroughton (2011)

4. Sheldon Cohen, PhD, *Social Relationships and Health,* Carnegie Mellon University (2004)

5. Rollin McCraty, PhD, "Link Between Emotions and Health," Institute of HeartMath (2011)

6. Eckhart Tolle, *The Power of Now,* New World Library (2004)

7. Lee Berk, "Laugher Remains Good Medicine," *American Physiological Society, Science Daily,* (2009)

8. www.newsroom.ucla.edu/releases/tai-chi-beats-back-depression-199019

9. www.heartmath.org

10. www.tappingsolutionfoundation.org

11. www.naet.com

12. www.spiritualresponse.com/

Chapter 32 Meditation: A Path to Wellness

1. Wayne Dyer, PhD, *10 Secrets for Success and Inner Peace,* Hay House (2001)

2. Jon Kabat-Zinn, *Full Catastrophe Living: Using the Wisdom of Your Body and Mind to Face Stress, Pain and Illness,* Bantam Books (2013)

3. Dina Proctor, *Madly Chasing Peace: How I Went from Hell to Happy in Nine Minutes a Day*, Morgan James Publishing, (2013)

4. www.news.harvard.edu/gazette/story/2011/01/eight-weeks-to-a-better-brain/

5. www.google.com/search?q=types+of+meditation&oq&aqs=type=chrome

Chapter 33 Energy Medicine, Alternative Medicine, and Miracles

1. Donna Eden, *Energy Medicine: Balancing Your Body's Energies for Optimal Health, Joy and Vitality,* Penguin Group (2008)

2. Wayne Dyer MD, *The Power of Intention*, Hay House (2005)

3. Wayne Dyer, MD, *Wishes Fulfilled*: Mastering the Art of Manifesting, Hay House, (2013)

4. Jack Canfield, *The Key to Living the Law of Attraction*, Health Communications, Inc. (2007)

5. Esther Hicks and Jerry Hicks, *Ask and it is Given: Learning to Manifest Your Desires,* Hay House (2010)

6. Robert E Detzler, *Spiritual Response Therapy Dictionary*, Spiritual Response Association (2008)

7. Roger Jahnke, *The Healer Within,* Harper Collins (2007)

8. Marianne Williamson, *A Return to Love: References on the Principles of A Course in Miracles,* Harper Collins (1975)

9. www.spiritualresponse.com

10. www.accesslife.net

About the Authors

Angie Lambert is an Intuitive Life Coach who offers intuitive counseling to clients worldwide. She is certified as a Holistic Health Coach, energy coach, Quantum Touch practitioner, and Tai chi instructor. Angie has a seven-year-old daughter and they currently live in the San Francisco Bay Area.

Sheri Miller is a certified Holistic Health Coach, Speech/Language Therapist and credentialed teacher. She shares from her heart all that she has learned over the past 20 years of research, teaching and personal experience. She has facilitated groups in Mindful Eating, the Emotional Freedom Technique (EFT), guided meditation, and has led women's spiritual groups. Sheri has two grown sons and lives in the San Francisco Bay Area.

If you would like to connect with us or provide feedback about this book, contact Angie or Sheri by emailing them at:

angieklambert@gmail.com or sherijane@gmail.com.

Check out Sheri's blog at:

www.healthyandradiantwithin.com

We would love to hear from you!